EXERCISES FOR
BRAIN HEALTH

EXERCISES FOR
BRAIN HEALTH

William Smith

Foreword by Joseph S. Sobelman, M.D.

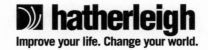

hatherleigh
Improve your life. Change your world.

Hatherleigh Press is committed to preserving and protecting the natural resources of the Earth. Environmentally responsible and sustainable practices are embraced within the company's mission statement.

Hatherleigh Press is a member of the Publishers Earth Alliance, committed to preserving and protecting the natural resources of the planet while developing a sustainable business model for the book publishing industry.

This book was edited, designed and photographed in the village of Hobart, New York. Hobart is a community that has embraced books and publishing as a component of its livelihood. There are several unique bookstores in the village. For more information, please visit www.hobartbookvillage.com.

www.hatherleighpress.com

Library of Congress Cataloging-in-Publication Data is available.

ISBN 978-1-57826-316-5

Exercises for Brain Health is available for bulk purchase, special promotions, and premiums. For information on reselling and special purchase opportunities, call 1-800-528-2550 and ask for the Special Sales Manager.

Cover design by Heather Daugherty
Interior design by Nick Macagnone

10 9 8 7 6 5 4 3 2 1

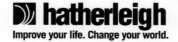

hatherleigh
Improve your life. Change your world.

DISCLAIMER

Consult your physician before beginning any exercise program. The author and publisher of this book and workout disclaim any liability, personal or professional, resulting from the misapplication of any of the following procedures described in this publication.

Table of Contents

FOREWORD

The United States is facing a demographic challenge. Our nation's population will "age rapidly when the Baby Boomers (people born between 1946 and 1964) begin to reach age 65 after the year 2010, [and] the percentage of the population aged 65 and over in the year 2050 is projected to be 20 percent" (*An Aging World*: 2008, U.S. Census Bureau).

The explosion of patients with conditions such as Alzheimer's disease, Parkinson's disease, and mild cognitive impairment account for a significant proportion of these statistics. Their impact is felt throughout all levels of society as individuals struggle with the associated memory loss, behavioral changes and problems performing activities of daily living.

In recent years, our understanding of the biology of aging, the genetic contribution to neurodegenerative diseases, and the physiology of dementia have increased dramatically. New techniques to image the brain, along with biomarkers to map susceptibility and novel therapies, have arisen as a result.

Perhaps even greater is our growing understanding of the importance of risk factor modification and lifestyle adjustments to assist patients and caregivers in their journey with dementia-related illnesses. It has now been widely proven that diet and exercise are key components in the management of such conditions

Exercises for Brain Health provides a valuable resource for people seeking guidance toward enhancing the mind-body connection via physical activity and motor stimulation. This book serves as an excellent outline for optimal achievement. Activities such as setting goals, structuring journals, and creating habits for healthy living are all described in simple language, making the critical decisions for cognitive improvement a realistic possibility. The need for this type of resource book has never been more relevant as Americans enter their golden years in ever increasing numbers.

Joseph S. Sobelman, M.D.
Neurologist

INTRODUCTION

Dementia: The Global Epidemic of Deteriorating Brain Function

If you are the loved one or a caregiver of an individual with dementia, you know how difficult managing this condition can be on you, your client or loved one, and their family. This book will help you improve your knowledge on how to effectively care for, and enhance quality of life, for those inflicted with deteriorating brain function.

You may have an elderly parent and are concerned about their long-term brain health, or maybe you intend to work as a health provider contracted for day-to-day care. This book will provide you with all you need to know to prevent brain deterioration, as well as give you warning signs so that you can treat symptoms promptly with therapeutic exercise, nutrition, and healthy brain exercises.

Dementia is not only prevalent in the United States but is actually frequently diagnosed across the globe. Developing and third world countries are undoubtedly being affected. However, without the medical technology to specifically target the nuances of the central nervous system (brain and spinal cord), cognitive function often goes unchecked. Instead, it is often assumed that memory loss, deterioration of language skills, motor skills problems, and decreasing brain function are normal in the aging process. Here's a wake-up call—they're not!

It is now estimated that 35 million people worldwide are living with Alzheimer's and other forms of brain-destroying diseases. The World Alzheimer Report estimates dementia will double every 20 years, thus affecting 115.4 million people worldwide by 2050. So what is the cause of this developing global epidemic? You might be surprised to find that several risk factors—including obesity, heart disease, poor nutrition, lack of physical activity, and diabetes—are at play. Individuals over 65 still tend to be the population most affected.

An initiative led by Alzheimer's Disease International projects 35.5 million by 2010 people will be diagnosed with dementia. The numbers breakdown as follows:

- 7 million in Western Europe
- 7 million in Asia
- 5.5 million in China
- 3 million in Latin America
- 5 million in U.S. (Alzheimer's Association)
- 1 in 8 people over 65 years
- 1 in 2 people over 85 years

Now the question is…how does exercise, nutrition, and practicing "brain games" decrease the likelihood that your loved ones will develop dementia? The following chapters will address this question, and much more.

CHAPTER ONE

Causes of Cognitive Disease

My first experience with dementia, specifically Alzheimer's, occurred when I was about 12 years old. Every year around the holidays, my family would travel to New Jersey to get together with my great-aunt and other members of the family. The year I was 12, I noticed for the first time that my great-aunt would demonstrate odd behaviors, tell unintelligible stories, and talk to herself at all hours of the night. I just couldn't understand why she talked to herself when no one else was in the room, or why she seemed delusional. As a loved one or caregiver of someone with dementia, you may have had an experience similar to this one. No matter whether you are an adult or a child, seeing someone with dementia for the first time can be a shock.

As I grew older, I learned that my great-aunt had Alzheimer's disease. This disease ultimately accounted for her depression, isolation from social activities, and a lack of executive functioning skills including basic cognition and daily living. As time went on, I came to experience similar scenarios, both professionally and personally, and my understanding of Alzheimer's and how it affects the lives of patients and their families has broadened significantly.

Today I now know that the Alzheimer's disease (AD) my great-aunt had is categorized as a primary dementia. Another form of primary dementia is called vascular dementia (VaD), an ischemic condition where blood flow and nutrients are slowly cut off from the tissues that need them, particularly in the brain. Vascular dementia is very similar in origin to another cerebral vascular condition called a stroke as both conditions involve decreased blood flow and oxygen to brain tissues. The fact is that dementia and stroke have parallels in which exercise can greatly benefit both conditions by improving cardiovascular and circulatory functions. Parkinson's disease (PD) is considered a secondary dementia.

What's the Difference Between Dementia and Cognitive Impairment?

Dementia literally means, "deprived mind." Cognitive impairment should be thought of differently from dementia because mild cognitive impairment does not transcend into dementia until daily activities are interrupted. In other words, dementia can be thought of as "severe cognitive impairment."

The good news is that dementia, a type of severe cognitive impairment, can be treated and controlled. Moreover, it presents in similar ways to other preventable diseases. Caregivers and loved ones to an elderly individual can be clued into the possibility of dementia by high blood pressure, decreased cardiovascular function, and overall increases in cardiovascular problems. These may lead to vascular dementia and an overall, gradual decline in physical and cognitive capabilities. Therefore, it is important to watch for the signs and act on them promptly. In the following sections, you will learn about the causes of dementia, the effects of dementia on the brain, how dementia is diagnosed, and how new hope is being offered for treatment.

Anatomy of Dementia

Dementia is caused by what takes place in the brain. A breakdown in the brain, in turn, effects the nervous system. The nervous system of an animal coordinates the activity of the muscles, monitors the organs, constructs (and also stops) input from the senses, and initiates actions. Prominent participants in the nervous system include neurons (also known as nerve cells), which play an important role in such coordination.

One of the most important components of the central nervous system is the brain. A human brain weighs approximately 3 pounds, and has 100 billion neurons that form a complex network of chemical and electrical communications. It's estimated that just one neuron may be connected to 100,000 additional neurons!

In the case of Alzheimer's the neural connections break down, slowing the speed of connections that contribute to communication, reasoning, and interpersonal socialization.

Neurons
As explained above, neurons are vitally important in the communication between the brain and the rest of the body. A neuron is comprised of three main parts: the cell body, dendrites and axons. The diagram below shows an example of each component of a neuron:

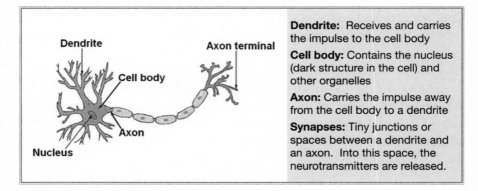

Dendrite: Receives and carries the impulse to the cell body

Cell body: Contains the nucleus (dark structure in the cell) and other organelles

Axon: Carries the impulse away from the cell body to a dendrite

Synapses: Tiny junctions or spaces between a dendrite and an axon. Into this space, the neurotransmitters are released.

Clumps of protein called tangled fibers can sometimes develop inside neurons, resulting in plaque deposits that interrupt nerve conductivity. These 'clumps' hinder the interaction of various neurotransmitters including acetylcholine, which helps to form memories. Similarly, reduced levels of endorphins have been linked to the development of Parkinson's. The good news is that endorphins can be stimulated through exercise, helping to prevent the onset of this disease.

Peripheral Nervous System

The peripheral nervous system can be thought of as the branches of a tree, in relation to the central nervous system. Picture the brain as the trunk of this tree with hundreds, even thousands, of branches (neurons) reaching out. Now imagine each branch is transmitting signals to an adjacent branch–that's essentially how neurons work! When dementia sets in, changes take place that decrease the speed and quality of how nerves and brain tissue works.

Remember:

Be sure to practice the Techniques on pages 66-68 with your patient or loved one every day to improve brain health!

Where and How the Brain is Effected by Dementia

The basal ganglia and cerebellum are two areas in the brain that modify movement on a minute-to-minute basis. Health professionals that work with persons stricken with dementia realize they must have an understanding of where and how this disease effects movement and cognition. Parkinson's, a secondary form of dementia, very often presents the person with physical movement challenges whereas Alzheimer's will present more often in limitations on cognitive functions, including memory. This is a very important point because it means that Parkinson's patients have full cognitive awareness of their dysfunction, while Alzheimer's patients generally do not. Thus, the balance between the basal ganglia and cerebellum allows for smooth, coordinated movement, and a disturbance in either system will show up as movement disorders. Caregivers must recognize physical activity is vital for physical functioning, particularly for Parkinson's patients.

To the right is a diagram depicting the cerebellum and its interaction with the motor center, or "action center," of the brain. Disruption in this loop between the brain and body will cause imbalance, trouble with coordination, and difficulty walking. Symptoms seen in Parkinson's may also include tremors or swaying of the body.

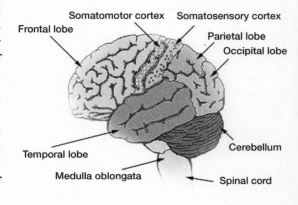

4

What the Studies Say

How is dementia diagnosed, and what causes it? The brain and spinal cord, the primary areas of the body impacted by Alzheimer's and Parkinson's, are enclosed in a hard skull and a protective vertebral column, respectively. Without current technology, we would not be able to access these areas in order to obtain an effective analysis. Now, as technology advances, accessibility to these areas provides greater opportunities and more significant depths of study, allowing doctors to more accurately diagnose dementia and leading to conclusions about dementia's possible causes.

The sub-specialty neuroradiology, a combination of neurology (study of the nervous system) and radiology (a diagnostic specialty), uses many of the newest scanning technologies to diagnose lesions, deterioration of nerve conductivity, and deep brain dysfunction. Corresponding advances in technology and medical research (such as the 320-slice CT scan, which allows for full brain imaging at half the radiation exposure) allow for major advancements in diagnostic care.

As we will discuss in the following chapters, a confirmed diagnosis of Alzheimer's is not conclusive until an autopsy of the brain is performed. However, cutting-edge research is fueling potential diagnostic tools to assist in patient care without the need for an autopsy.

Among these assessment tools are new blood serum tests to diagnose Alzheimer's. Clinical validations of these blood tests are currently ongoing, but private industry has found diagnostic results for AD-specific blood markers to be 95 percent accurate.

In addition to blood tests, scans are being developed that are capable of directly measuring brain activity. At New York University, researchers are using electroencephalogram (EEG) scans to determine normal brain waves versus ones that may eventually lead to a form of dementia. The EEG is being utilized to develop software that will differentiate abnormal versus normal right/left brain activity, thereby indicating the likelihood of developing early onset dementia. Leslie Prichep, an associate director of the Brain Research Laboratories of the Department of Psychiatry at New York University School of Medicine, notes that their EEG method is nearly 95 percent accurate in distinguishing between those who would decline in terms of brain function and those who would not. The theta brain wave (which originates in a region of the brain shown to be impaired in dementia patients) is much more prominent in people likely to exhibit mental decline. Prichep says this is important to detect because drugs are now becoming available, which can lessen or eliminate the development of dementia. With tests like the EEG, patients can determine whether they are at higher risk of developing dementia, and can then take specific drugs in order to slow, or completely stop, their mental decline. Moreover, this new technique is less expensive, less painful and less invasive than using traditional MRIs to evaluate brain function.

CHAPTER TWO

Types of Cognitive Disease

Perhaps the most important fact for any loved one or caregiver of an elderly individual to remember is this:

Although it is common in very elderly individuals,
dementia is not a normal part of the aging process.

In other words, we can take steps to lower the odds of dementia affecting someone we care for.

The National Institute of Neurological Disorders and Stroke (NINDS) describes dementia as follows: "Dementia is not a specific disease. It is a descriptive term for a collection of symptoms that can be caused by a number of disorders that affect the brain."

As outlined in the previous chapter, effects of dementia on the brain include problems with cognitive ability (problem-solving, memory), behavioral ability (social agitation, delusions), and physical activities. Inhibited brain function causes a severe impact on basic independence, mobility, and daily functioning. This has an effect on those living with or caring for the person afflicted with dementia. For those suffering from dementia, daily activities, and even simple tasks such as bathing, conversation, dressing, navigating stairs, and walking around the block, become increasingly difficult. On the whole, life for those with dementia is unmanageable without care from loved ones or caregivers.

This book helps in providing strategies to manage activities of daily living including bathing, dressing, walking, and stair climbing, with greater ease.

Primary Dementia: Alzheimer's Disease

Alzheimer's disease is a form of primary dementia and, most often, this is the form of dementia you hear about in the media, along with Parkinson's.

Often, as with many other diseases, Alzheimer's patients are not necessarily aware they have the disease.

Alzheimer's disease (AD) is named after Alois Alzheimer, the German doctor who first described how it impacts various cognitive (decision-making capabilities) and chronic physical conditions. The National Institute of Aging (NIA) notes that Alzheimer's "attacks parts of the brain that control memory (hippocampus), language/reasoning, and ultimately may lead to unresponsiveness to the outside world." The inherent nature of Alzheimer's is degeneration; that is, as the disease progresses, normal activity becomes more and more difficult.

In Alzheimer's disease, neurons (the functional cell that allows transmission of chemical and electrical brain signals) are lost in large numbers, impacting basic functions in the brain.

The NIA provides three major characteristics of a brain with Alzheimer's disease: Amyloid plaques, neurofibrillary tangles, and an inflammatory state (oxidative breakdown, catabolic state). Loss of connections between neurons can result in neural cell death, thereby affecting basic human processes including reasoning, language skills, and social interaction.

Plaques (Beta-amyloids) are found outside neurons (nerve cells), whereas neurofibrillary tangles are found within neurons. Both plaques and tangles are found in brains without Alzheimer's disease, yet are found in extraordinarily large amounts in those with the disease.

Generally, Alzheimer's disease is broken down into two types: early-onset and late-onset. The NIA notes that early-onset Alzheimer's disease occurs most frequently in people with a family history and can manifest itself as early as their thirties. More than 90 percent of Alzheimer's cases are late-onset and develop in people older than 60. Late-onset Alzheimer's is emphasized in this book because genetic, environmental, and lifestyle factors are typically to blame when the disease occurs later in life. This book focuses on social and lifestyle factors, thereby targeting late on-set Alzheimer's, yet with appropriate early intervention strategies, those with signs of early cognitive decline can benefit as well.

Remember:
Be sure to practice the Techniques on pages 66-68 with your patient or loved one every day to improve brain health!

Diagnosing Alzheimer's Disease
Identifying those at risk for Alzheimer's early on is vital in providing therapeutic treatments, including drugs, exercise, social support systems, and cognitive intelligence building strategies. However, a diagnosis of Alzheimer's is not absolute. Alzheimer's disease can only be conclusively diagnosed upon death with an autopsy of the brain. In a living patient, if Alzheimer's disease is suspected by family or loved ones, a medical professional (such as a neurologist) will take an extensive medical history, perform the necessary physical exam, and test skills related to memory, language, and brain function. Diagnostically speaking, these are the only 'tools' available to diagnose AD, since the specific area of the brain affected by Alzheimer's disease cannot be viewed in a living patient. NINDS notes the diagnosis of dementia is generally made if two or more brain functions are affected: memory and language, for example.

A diagnosis of Alzheimer's is generally confirmed through three different methods: individual and family history, memory tests, and scans (MRI, PET, CT, and EEG). These methods are effective but not absolute. Since these scans have only recently become available, the understanding and treatment methods of Alzheimer's and dementia have grown by leaps and bounds in a short amount of time.

Primary Dementia: Vascular Dementia

Although Alzheimer's is the most prevalent cause of dementia, vascular dementia comes in at a close second and can be just as debilitating. As much as 20 percent of all dementias are caused by vascular dementia and is a direct result of brain damage induced by strokes and other assorted cerebrovascular or cardiovascular problems.

Vascular dementia can be closely compared to cardiovascular disease, namely heart and vascular disease. When we think of heart disease, the image of cholesterol clogging arteries and raising blood pressure comes to mind. Coincidentally, these are symptoms of hypertension, which is a risk factor for developing dementia. In the case of vascular dementia, the term "ischemia" (the slow choking off of oxygen to vital brain structures) is often thought of in a similar context. This results in slowing of brain processes, inability to concentrate, and over the long-term a toxic, inflammatory environment develops around living tissues. Oftentimes, inflammation can lead to "oxidative stress" that fosters a pro-inflammatory environment, which proves to be very bad for healthy living tissue. Imagine a really bad case of indigestion, but in your brain!

The inflammatory process affects oxidation, which is vital to how cells breathe. During oxidation, by-products are created called 'pro-oxidants'. These pro-oxidants damage cells and initiate the inflammatory process. How do we combat the unwanted by-products of inflammation? By eating foods nutritionally rich in anti-oxidants including dark vegetables, colorful fruits, nuts, whole grains, garlic, and soy.

As mentioned earlier, vascular dementia has many similar risk factors to cardiovascular disease, one of which is inflammation. It has been found that "visceral fat," or belly fat, is linked to pro-inflammatory states. Other shared risk factors include genetic pre-disposition (parents' body types), improper diet, lack of exercise, and excessive calorie intake. In addition, decreasing calorie intake, or "calorie restriction," has been shown to prevent many chronic medical conditions, in addition to cardiovascular disease and dementia.

Secondary Dementia: Parkinson's Disease

Whereas Alzheimer's tends to be characterized by cognitive impairment, Parkinson's commonly presents itself more overtly during movement and therefore belongs to a group of conditions called "movement disorders". Seemingly simple movements (including walking) become difficult, muscles suffer rigid contractions, and facial expressions may become unexpressive.

Muhammad Ali, Michael J. Fox, Janet Reno, Pope John Paul II, and Salvador Dali are notable figures that have this debilitating condition. Life with Parkinson's, as Michael J. Fox discusses in his documentary, *Always Looking Up: The Adventures of an Incurable Optimist,* can be both physically and emotionally fatiguing.

Risk Factors of Parkinson's Disease

Identifying risk factors for Parkinson's, as with any disease, is half the battle. Risk factors include:

Aging process: While aging is a risk factor, growing older does not mean someone is pre-destined for Parkinson's and/or conditions related to dementia.

Gender: Males are more likely than females to develop Parkinson's.

Family history (genetic predisposition): Heredity, although small, does play a part in one's risk for developing Parkinson's. Find out if there you have a family history of Parkinson's or other dementia-related illnesses.

Chemical exposure: Exposure to chemicals including pesticides or herbicides.

Inadequate levels of B vitamin folate: Nutritional deficiencies including inadequate levels of vitamin B folate have been cited as risk factors for developing Parkinson's. Make sure your client or loved one has their blood work profile updated annually.

Incidental tremors, decreased motor control, and twitching are only three physical symptoms of this disease that are formed by chemical imbalances. Other symptoms include muscle rigidity, a slowing of physical movement (bradykinesia) and, in extreme cases, a loss of physical movement (akinesia). These primary symptoms are the result of decreased stimulation of the motor cortex by the basal ganglia (see Chapter 1), normally caused by the insufficient formation and action of dopamine, which is produced in the dopaminergic neurons of the brain.

Secondary symptoms may include high level cognitive dysfunction and subtle language problems. Additionally, Parkinson's is characterized by a masked, or non-expressive, face, decrease in voice power, writing in tiny letters, drooling, slow movements, and small, yet distinct, at-rest tremors.

Occurring in 1 of 300 people, Parkinson's is a progressive, degenerative disease that gets worse with time. Persons with this condition have a fully intact cerebrum, yet a greatly impaired central nervous system. Worse yet, whereas Alzheimer's patients may not be aware that they have the condition, those stricken with Parkinson's are fully aware they have disease.

CHAPTER THREE

Understanding the Signs and Symptoms of Cognitive Disease

Now that we've covered the three most commonly diagnosed types of dementias, let's move on to discuss the basics of how dementia impacts the body as well as typical human behavior. Often, it is changes in demeanor and physical ability that alert family and friends to the possibility that a loved one may have dementia. Diagnosing and treating the condition as early as possible is key to alleviating the impact of dementia and the effects that it's symptoms will have on quality of life.

The signs and symptoms of dementia are wide-ranging and can be easily recognized by loved ones and caregivers. Dementia may sometimes become apparent with the slowing of cognitive functions as in Alzheimer's, or with movement difficulties as commonly seen in Parkinson's.

Many times, the signs and symptoms of dementia vary and cannot be easily categorized as either physical or mental decline. In these cases, symptoms may appear to be both physical and mental. Utilizing an assessment tool, such as the one below, can be very helpful in observing and interacting with your loved one and can help your medical provider in providing the best treatment by providing valuable information.

Common Signs and Symptoms of Dementia:

- **Forgetfulness:** immediate recall memory may be affected, but over time long-term memory may also be diminished.
- **Disorientation:** having trouble determining one's surroundings, for example becoming confused when finding the way back home from a local store or a daily walk.
- **Trouble with everyday tasks:** this may include administering daily medications, preparing breakfast, etc.
- **Personality changes:** ranges of irritability, for example an outwardly expressive person may become a very quiet, introverted person.

Checklist for Noting Symptoms in Dementia Patients

The list below can be used by family members and friends of patients with dementia. For each, note the current condition of your loved one. This will help you better evaluate their daily progress and can also be very informative for their medical provider.

Physical health: incontinence, difficulty with balance and walking, frequent falls, nutrition, dental, hearing, vision, sexual functioning

Mental Health: cognitive function, depression, anxiety

Functioning: basic activities of daily living (includes feeding, walking, dressing, bathing, getting out of bed, and grooming), instrumental activities of daily living (includes using the telephone, shopping, food preparation, laundry, managing medications, and managing finances)

Social support: caregiver burden, finances, communication, possibility of any abuse and/or neglect

Environmental adequacy: safety of surroundings, health issues due to climate

Alzheimer' Symptoms

Loved ones and caregivers that recognize the signs and symptoms of dementia can be of great help in treatment, particularly in the case of conditions such as Alzheimer's where symptoms sometimes progress slowly. Below are common signs for recognizing Alzheimer's:

- Forgetting recently learned information
- Difficulty with problem solving capacities, for example calculating one's check book
- Difficulty completing common tasks at home including daily household chores
- Disorientation with time or place
- Trouble with spatial and visual images
- Poor decision-making capabilities
- Withdrawal from social or work activities
- Erratic personality shifts such as depression, anxiety, or confused states

According to John B. Arden, Ph. D., director of training for psychology at Kaiser Permanente Medical Centers in Northern California, you should make your medical provider aware of the following signs if they persist in a loved one:

- They repeatedly get lost on a familiar route.
- They have difficulty finding words to express themselves.
- They are unable to identify common objects.
- At times, they don't know where they are or what time of day it is.
- They ask the same question over and over when they're not trying to get a different answer.

CHAPTER FOUR

Maintaining a Healthy Brain for Years to Come

Wе often overlook the importance of lifestyle (for example, nutrition and exercise) when it comes to brain health. In the following chapter, we will discuss some of the many lifestyle factors that can impact one's likelihood of developing dementia and how you can help your loved one to control these factors and obtain a better quality of life.

We often associate the stress response in the body to work or family activities that place us in situations that are not quick or pleasant. The stress response, also known as 'fight-or-flight,' can also be caused by poor nutritional intake. Suboptimal nutritional intake leads to increased acidity in the blood, chemical and hormonal imbalances, and ultimately an acidic environment that destroys neurons in the brain. The fight-or-flight response is notorious for stimulating the adrenal glands and ultimately cortisol release, intimately linked to imbalances in blood acidity

So how do we create the nurturing, nutrient rich environment that fosters healthy brain tissue?

Calorie Restriction Decreases the Risk of Disease

Seventy years ago, research suggested that calorie restriction was linked to prevention of various chronic diseases including heart disease, diabetes and Alzheimer's disease. These conditions are generally age-related, not age-dependent. In other words, it should not be assumed that these ailments will afflict an individual simply because they have reached a certain age. Alzheimer's, for example, affects geriatric populations but is not a normal part of aging. Recent research has linked reducing caloric intake to prevention. Now, we have a unique opportunity to prevent certain dementia-like diseases. This means that reducing caloric intake is key to taking an active role in preventing these diseases.

The Evidence

The connection between calorie restriction and disease prevention has been studied for over 50 years and the evidence remains relevant today. Scientists have discovered that when animals are forced to live on 30% to 40% fewer calories than they would normally consume, they become resistant to most age-related diseases and live 30% to 50% longer. It's easy to see how this research is potentially relevant to humans. Like the mice in these studies, many of us are middle-aged mammals who eat a high-calorie, high-fat diet. While research results in mice do not always prove true in humans, this is often the case.

Calorie-restriction studies such as this demonstrate the many benefits of reducing calories and fat in one's diet. This is especially important for individuals with dementia, or those at risk of developing dementia, because consuming a lower-calorie diet has been shown to aid in preventing the onset of age-related diseases.

Hydration: Water Intake and Brain Health

Hydrate, Hydrate, Hydrate! 60% of our body is water. That means we should take in half our body weight, or 25-30% percent, through our diet. This is equivalent to 6-8 8 oz. glasses of water per day. Ask yourself, does the person you care for do this? Encourage him or her to drink water regularly by always having it nearby. Having bottled water on hand when traveling or on hand during physical activity will increase the likeliness of fluid intake.

Oddly enough, you should drink when you're not thirsty: this is because, by the time you experience thirst, your body has already been deprived of the hydration it needs for some time. Remember, don't let your loved one wait until they're parched to drink water; rather, encourage them to drink water before that occurs.

In addition, teach them to keep tabs on visible feedback including urine color, skin pliability, and normal sweating. Urine color should be pale to light in color. Skin pliability should stretch and return to normal texture immediately. Sweating can be an additional indication of proper hydration. Sweating during exercise and physical activity is normal and expected. Exercise without sweating, while it does happen, is not a regular occurrence.

> The human body is made of 60% water, and the brain 80%. The brain, spinal cord, nervous, blood, and every other important piece of body anatomy relies heavily on water, or the fluids it makes up such as cerebrospinal fluid (CSP). Our brains sit in CSP that bathes, lubricates, cushions, and hydrates the convoluted folds of the brain itself.

The Danger of Dehydration
Difficulty concentrating, fatigue, and stiffness in body tissues may be caused by dehydration. The general recommendation is 6-8 glasses of water per day, yet with elderly populations this amount is easily decreased by 1-2 glasses. Low hydration is a concern even in inactive populations that do not physically exert themselves beyond activities of daily living. Basic physiological functions including digestion, perspiration, urination, and renal function all require fluids.

Decreasing Inflammation: Free radicals, Antioxidants, and Aging of our Cells
Many of us have heard the term inflammation, but what exactly is it? The body's pH is the measurement of alkalinity or acidity in the body's biochemistry, specifically the fluid environments such as blood or spinal fluid that exist throughout the body. The key is to find a balance in the body between the necessary acidity found in the stomach, for example, while keeping low acidity in the intestine and blood.

Factors that contribute to inflammation:
- **Stress:** Good (eustress) or Bad (distress)
- **Inadequate or erratic sleep patterns**
- **Poor nutrition:** trans/saturated fats, processed foods, refined carbohydrates

19

- **Diuretics:** Drinking excess soda, tea/coffee, water pills
- **Food supply chain:** genetically modified foods, hormone injected animals/foods
- **Environment:** Urban areas, smog-centric geography
- **Medications**

Strategies to stabilize pH and decrease long-term inflammatory diseases (such as cancer):

- **Consume a variety of colorful fruits and vegetables**—favor dark, leafy vegetables
- **Drink 6-10 glasses of fluid** (water, natural juices, dark teas)
- **Favor non-red meat sources, including fish**
- **Good fats include Omega 3's, 6's, deep-water fatty fishes, flax seeds, and nuts**
- **Do not overcook foods:** This de-natures, or breaks down, the protein bond and makes the food source more unstable before it enters the body

Concentration of Hydrogen ions compared to distilled water		Examples of solutions at this pH
10,000,000	pH=0	Battery Acid, Strong Hydrofluoric Acid
1,000,000	pH=1	Hydrochloric Acid Secreted by Stomach Lining
100,000	pH=2	Lemon Juice, Gastric Acid, Vinegar
10,000	pH=3	Grapefruit, Orange Juice, Soda
1,000	pH=4	Acid Rain, Tomato Juice
100	pH=5	Soft Drinking Water, Black Coffee
10	pH=6	Urine, Saliva
1	pH=7	"Pure" Water
1/10	pH=8	Sea Water
1/100	pH=9	Baking Soda
1/1,000	pH=10	Great Salt Lake, Milk of Magnesia
1/10,000	pH=11	Ammonia Solution
1/100,000	pH=12	Soapy Water
1/1,000,000	pH=13	Bleaches, Oven Cleaner
1/10,000,000	pH=14	Liquid Drain Cleaner

Antioxidants work to deter the impact of oxidants that contribute to cellular aging (i.e. aging, brain death, and basically getting old!). Vitamins E, C, and A have been touted as antioxidants, too.

How do you control the damaging impact of inflammation?
- Light therapy (see page 31)
- Nutrition
- Sleep

Have You Heard of the Following Nutrient Terms?

Folate, Omega-3, simple sugars, refined foods Vitamin C, Vitamin B Complex (B1, B6, and B12), Zinc, multi-vitamins.

B-vitamins have been linked to forgetfulness and accelerated periods of forgetfulness outside of the natural progression of aging. Aging can be defined as the natural biological and physiological process of cell aging, yet the process can be slowed significantly and function improved on both mental and physical levels.

Following a high fiber, lean protein, whole-grain, and anti-inflammatory diet is key to brain health.

The Integrative Medicine Program at the Atlantic Health System in New Jersey provides very specific guidelines to apply to day-to-day healthy brain nutritional intake:

- Avoid high-fructose corn syrups and simple or additive sugared foods as much as possible. Sugar is poison to brain and blood, as exemplified by the connection between diabetes and dementia.
- Cold-water fatty fish, flaxseeds, walnuts, and beans like navy, kidney, and soy are all great sources of Omega-3's. Studies have shown that 1-2 servings of Omega-3 rich fish per week decreases the risk for Alzheimer's disease. Serving size is 3 oz or roughly the size of a deck of cards.

Fruits, Vegetables, and Colorful Foods
Natural foods, basically anything unprocessed from the ground and raised organically, is great. Trust me, organic foods are not the only way to go, but if there's an option between foods raised with pesticides or genetically-modified, it's in your loved one's best interest to pursue the least chemically-laced product.

Fiber, antioxidants, and phytochemicals are in plentiful supply in dark leafy vegetables, red peppers, spaghetti squash, bean varieties, and electrolyte-rich bananas. Bananas are also high in B vitamins that support the nervous system.

Atlantic Health System notes 200 students at a Twickenham (Middlesex) school were helped through their exams this year by eating bananas at breakfast, break, and lunch in a bid to boost their brainpower. Research has shown that the potassium-packed fruit can assist learning by making pupils more alert.

Building a Better Brain

Brain health in the elderly, or any age for that matter, is a hot button topic. Forgetting where they placed their keys or questioning if they turned off the lights are common, everyday concerns. Yet does this happen everyday to them? Have they recently forgotten how to get home from the job they've worked at for 20 years?

The Population Reference Bureau indicates that 1 in 12 elderly people experience a decline in cognitive function so severe they have difficulty performing the normal activities of daily living, and eventually, cannot live independently. Imagine your family member is one that needs assistance; this changes your life immediately.

Yet the decline of brain health, or cognitive decline, doesn't have to be a normal part of aging.

Researcher Kenneth Langa at the University of Michigan School of Medicine and Institute for Social Research found that education level seems to be a determinant in cognitive health as we age. Langa concluded that individuals with higher levels of education are at a lesser risk of suffering cognitive decline. Keeping your brain sharp by continuing to learn—no matter what your education level—is always important to preventing the onset of dementia.

Continuing to learn and build the "buff brain" we all want is possible, and should be part of our effort towards healthy living. New studies that focus around fancy names like 'neuroplasticity' and 'neurogenesis,' essentially study how the brain deforms and learns based upon new stimuli by connecting new connections between neurons. This is great news because a lot of this positive research on brain health points to exercise as the key.

Remember:
Be sure to practice the Techniques on pages 66-68 with your
patient or loved one every day to improve brain health!

Develop a Social Support System for the Patient:
Supporting the Caregiver

Companionship and connectedness with one's surroundings is vital to those
with dementia or dementia-like symptoms. Having a support system (for
example, a dependable neighbor or a family member) in place so the patient
can receive assistance in activities such as administration of daily medications
or performing daily exercises is especially important in enhancing the quality
of life for those with dementia.

Does your loved one need help with their health?
- Have they experienced a recent dramatic weight loss?
- Is the home still a safe place for them to be alone?
- Are they still independent?
- Has their health changed in recent years?

Dementia is a progressive condition, and the responsibility of caring for a
loved one can often last for many years. This takes its toll on the physical,
emotional, and mental health of both the caregiver and the person afflicted.
If you are currently caring for a loved one with dementia and feel a need to
establish a greater support system, don't wait. Friends, family members,
community members and church organizations are just a few examples of
resources to explore.

Similarly, healthy living is important for both the caregiver and the afflicted
person. This includes reaching out to others for additional support when
needed, staying organized with to-do lists, and paying close attention to your
own stress levels.

Visit the Resources section on page 146 for more information on helpful
resources for caregivers and loved ones of dementia patients.

The Alzheimer's Association is an excellent resource for locating on-line,
community, and clinical support. For example, say you are considering
placing a family member in assisted living because they've fallen several
times in the last month and are not safe at home anymore. Preparing

Medicare/Medicaid documents, senior living options, and 24/7 questions become increasingly important questions. These questions can change daily, yet the Internet has created an informed generation with information at our fingertips.

Caregivers should have a daily, weekly, and monthly schedule of activities for the patient. This list of priorities may be spread over family members and friends to prevent caregiver burnout.

Daily Examples:	Weekly Examples:	Monthly Examples:
• Medicines • Bathing • Physical activity: therapeutic exercise • Cognitive activity: reading the paper, playing Chess • Change of environments: grocery store, shopping	• Doctors' visits • Activities in community • Family visits	• Plan a ½ day or day trip • Restocking of medications • Educational opportunities: concerts, opera, book readings

Creating A Social Support System

Establishing a network of close relationships for a dementia patient is an excellent strategy that will support the physical and mental exercises contained in the Programs in Chapter 8.

Getting out of the house and meeting people should be the first step. Opening up the world of a person stricken with dementia by meeting other people will completely change their outlook on life. We know that isolation from others can lead to depression, which compounds dementia-like symptoms. Those endorphins (a.k.a. the body's natural pain medication) are released through fulfilling, happy experiences. By engaging friendly and caring individuals, the person with dementia reinforces the healthy neural connections and creates new ones.

Communicating feelings and emotions openly between family and a person with dementia is often difficult yet necessary. Listening can often be the most important skill a caregiver demonstrates. Non-verbal communication patterns from someone with dementia including abnormal lethargy, withdrawal from

For caregivers, help your patient or loved one get their day back on track with these 10 tips that will help smooth out the ups and downs in their daily schedule:

1. Stretch for 5 minutes before getting out of bed in the morning to prepare your muscles for movement.

2. Lay your clothes out for the next day prior to going to bed. Confusion is common first thing in the morning as the optic nerve and ocular muscles around the eyes have been in a state of relaxation throughout the night, so chances are that matching clothes will not be an easy task to perform in the morning.

3. Drink one large glass of water in the morning to stabilize your morning eating habits. Our bodies are approximately 60% water. By replenishing our body first thing in the morning, the regulatory systems of our body, namely heart rate and blood pressure, will stay increasingly balanced.

4. Eat 300-400 calories for breakfast. Research has shown that eating breakfast improves memory performance.

5. Healthy lunch foods can easily be made to order at local restaurants. Pick steamed and broiled foods over fried. Gastro-Intestinal (GI) irritability can be exacerbated by fried and processed foods.

6. Mid-afternoon is a perfect time to have a moderate carbohydrate/moderate protein-based snack or drink. An example would be a smoothie of dark berries with whey protein blended with water. Martha Raidl, a nutrition specialist at the University of Idaho Extension Program suggests beverages like plain or flavored water, or iced or hot tea as long as it's unsweetened. If this doesn't satisfy you, try a 100-calorie snack.

7. Early dinners around 5:00 or 6:00 can be on the heavier side, whereas dinners at 7:00 or later should be on the lighter side. If you know your dinner will be later, add another serving of milk instead of water to your smoothie, increasing the total caloric intake for your mid-afternoon snack.

8. Take a walk after dinner, but wait 20-30 minutes after eating. Stimulating blood flow through aerobically-based movements that are low impact (not running) aids in the digestive process. Giving 30 minutes allows the food to settle.

9. Write a short to-do list before going to bed. Keep your list to 3 priority items if you do not work and 1-2 priority items if you have a full-time occupation.

10. Practice deep breathing as a form of relaxation before bed. Deep breathing is an excellent way to slow the heart rate. Focus on breathing in through the nose and out through the mouth.

normally enjoyable activities, and forgetting names of loved ones are not only risk factors, but also signs the disease is progressing.

For Loved Ones: Establishing Your Network of Professional Caregivers

In addition to friends and family, professionals that have extensive experience and knowledge-based intellect in the field of dementia are vital. This is hardly an all-inclusive list, so please refer to your primary care provider for additional information.

Primary Care Physician
Primary care practitioners are coming back into vogue. The "medical home" model, in which the emphasis lies on a personal physician in a long-term medical relationship with the patient thus capable of acute, chronic and continuous and comprehensive care, is re-empowering the original provider of medical care. The trend over the last couple of decades has drifted away from the primary care doctor towards specialists that order expensive tests and scans. Having one point of contact is key to coordinating patient care.

Neurologist
Neurologists are doctors that work with the nervous system and assessing its function. A neurologist is likely the medical provider that will provide the most clinical care to someone with dementia.

Psychologist or Psychiatrist
The mental aspects of dementia are too exhaustive to mention here. Knowing that the mental and physical aspects of dementia are substantive, having a healthcare professional on your dementia-support team is vital.

Social Worker
An experienced social worker can coordinate family and friends, along with the necessary medical care. Social workers become an integral part of the familial structure when there has been an injury or acute medical incident (stroke, fall, etc.) that has led to the one suffering with dementia to become disabled.

Physical and/or Occupational Therapist
Clinical rehabilitation (pain free, range of motion) and restoring function are the PT or OTs' initial objectives. Their next goal is to establish an exercise program that can be taken with the patient following treatment.

Fitness Professional (i.e. Personal Trainer)
As a physical trainer, this category is dear to my heart! The personal trainer is the frontline of prevention. Listening, interpersonal communication skills, and knowledge-based skills are absolutes for quality personal trainers. Solid trainers have an excellent repertoire with medical providers and colleagues in the fitness community.

In addition to the traditional approach of care as stated, Johns Hopkins in 2009 introduced a new model for emerging Alzheimer's care called "Habilitation." Habilitation focuses on respecting the feelings of people with Alzheimer's and making the most of their remaining capacities, rather than trying to restore lost abilities (rehabilitation)—often in vain—or impose rigid standards for thoughts and behavior. Habilitation encourages caregivers to connect with patients on an emotional level rather than argumentatively getting them to agree with the fact that he or she has lost a loved one or cannot accomplish the same daily activities they used to before the illness.

This book also encourages caregivers to pursue interaction with those afflicted with dementia diseases by engaging them emotionally through activities he or she enjoys, particularly physical activities in a fitness professionals' care.

Finding the Needed Professionals to Work with Dementia Conditions

Adult Day Services Provider
Adult day services provide a variety of community-oriented settings that emphasize the social experience overseen by complimentary health and caregiver professionals. These day service centers provide socially uplifting activities during normal business hours. Many day services offer transportation, meals, snacks, personal care, and therapeutic activities.

Home-Based Care Services
Similar to adult day services in scope of practice, home-based care services may provide a cost-effective option to institutional care. Healthcare systems may offer this type of outreach program as an outpatient service or outsource to an outside contractor. Services may include 24-hour monitoring care, therapeutic services, daily activities that include grocery shopping or filling prescriptions, and cooking.

Independent Living Facilities
My maternal grandparents live in an independent living facility. These facilities have 24-hour services, medical response on-site including nurses

during scheduled times, and dining facilities. Private pay and subsidized-care is generally available through state and federal government housing authorities.

Assisted Living Residential Care

Assisted living care is the fastest growing segment of geriatric and senior populations. Daily activities including bathing, washing, cooking, and dressing are provided for the resident. Closer hands-on services are provided because of the level of disability or low-functioning of its residents.

Is an independent living facility right for your situation? How about if you're a child looking to place a parent? Have the person you're caring for check out the following checklists from Alternatives for Seniors (Summer/Fall 2009 Edition) to find out. If they answer yes to a majority of the following questions, an independent living facility might be right for them.

	Yes	Indifferent	No
I want to remain independent			
I have concerns about my health			
Emergency medical help is important to me			
Housekeeping assistance would be helpful to me			
I would like assistance with home maintenance and repairs			
I would enjoy the opportunity to meet new people in a social setting			
I would like assistance with some outdoor maintenance			
I would like planned social and recreational activities			
I would like transportation service available			
I would like meals prepared for me			

	Yes	Indifferent	No
I am willing to move from where I live now			
I am willing to have less living space in order to receive services such as prepared meals, maintenance, and housekeeping			
I would feel safer if I moved somewhere else			

Secondly, when visiting an independent living facility come prepared with the following observations and questions:

Observe the following:
- Activities (type and how frequently offered)
- Laundry facilities and services
- Scheduled transportation
- Emergency call system
- Staff available 24 hours/day
- Meals prepared to specific dietary requirements
- Housekeeping

When touring the facility ask yourself the following questions:
- Are Guest Suites available for overnight stays?
- Were current residents using the activity room?
- Were any residents using the exercise facilities?
- Are carpets and furniture clean?
- Was staff friendly and respectful?
- Did staff know residents by name?
- What percentage of the apartments have been rented and are occupied?
- Is the management staff experienced? Effective? Friendly?
- Does the facility have a good reputation in the community?

Sleep

Sleep is similar to medicine and can heal the brain

Sleep is becoming an endangered resource. We live busier and busier lives that motivate us to work harder and longer. Sleep deprivation has been linked to increased risk of cardiovascular risk factors, slower reflexes, and negative mental functioning in the brain.

The National Institutes of Health estimate 60 million Americans have insomnia frequently or for extended periods of time. The NIH indicates sleep problems affect virtually every aspect of day-to-day living including mood, mental alertness, work performance, and energy level.

Sleep deprivation has direct links to impairments in concentration, memory, and cognitive function. Sleep acts as medicine for the brain, healing brain tissue that is under constant stress, both good and bad. Think of the brain as a computer that must shut down and "re-boot." This allows for the downtime the body needs for rest, recovery, and stimulating the 5 stages of sleeping cycles culminating in Rapid Eye Movement (REM) and Non Rapid Eye Movement (NREM) sleep. For a very interesting discussion on the stages of sleep, visit The University of Washington's neuroscience section on sleep.

Sleep deprivation places the body into a slightly altered state that "amounts to, in essence, a cane or walker for your brain," says David Katz, M.D.

Research recommends we get between 7-8 hours/sleep every night. Is this realistic? We know that sleep and memory are intimately linked, but what if someone is not getting their daily dose? Drugs, herbal remedies, and sleep clinics are often recommended.

Simple steps to promote quality sleep include the following:
- Avoid stimulants such as caffeine, alcohol, and chocolates before bed
- I recommend scheduling the most vigorous workouts earlier in the day
- As with dementia, repetition in activities is very important. Try to go to bed every night at the same time, take naps at regular intervals, and avoid sleeping during the day if you truly are not tired

Light Therapy: Daily Doses of UV Light

Light therapy has been used to heal tissues, treat Seasonal Affective Disorder (SAD), and decrease blood toxicity (i.e. alkalinity).

Natural light and artificially produced light (i.e. UV light) are both therapeutic in their own right. Natural light is excellent for stimulating vitamin D and enhancing calcium uptake for stronger bones. This is very important for geriatric populations. The use of UV is great for those living in cold climates or people with mental disorders including depression, another risk factor for dementia often associated with Alzheimer's.

Light therapy detoxifies the blood by altering the pH levels in the body. Cells break down when the environment they live in (for example, blood or cerebrospinal fluid) becomes increasingly acidic due to disease, poor nutrition, or chemical exposure. Light therapy, as simple as it may seem, can have a profound effect on reversing the effects of an aging body.

Depression and its Impacts Upon Mental and Physical Health

Dementia and depression often co-exist because high levels of cortisol (a marker of inflammation) may be associated with depression, and indeed stress, and may also cause neuronal death. Dementia is associated with nerves dying in the brain and ultimately causing physical and mental disability, visually present in conditions such as Parkinson's and Alzheimer's.

Social isolation has a significant impact upon mental and physical health, and should be classed among smoking and obesity as a major risk factor to health.

Stress Relievers: Breathing, Meditation, and Visual Imagery

Controlling risk factors including stress allows the body to fully realize the full benefit of regular physical activities. One method time and time again that has been shown to enhance mental acuity, focus, and brain function are "mind-body" connection exercises.

A Breathing Exercise: The Gateway to Daily Meditation

Focusing on the breath is one of the most common and fundamental techniques for accessing the meditative state. Breath is a deep rhythm of the body that connects us intimately with the world around us. Learn these steps, and then share them with someone you care for.

Close your eyes, breathe deeply and regularly, and observe your breath as it flows in through the nose and out of the mouth. Give your full attention to the breath as it comes in, and full attention to the breath as it goes out. Store your breath in the belly, not the chest, between inhales and exhales. Whenever you find your attention wandering away from your breath, gently pull it back to the rising and falling of the breath via the belly.

Inhale through your nose slowly and deeply, feeling the lower chest and abdomen inflate like a balloon. Hold for five seconds. Exhale deeply, deflating the lower chest and abdomen like an emptying balloon. Hold for five seconds. Do this 5 times, and then allow your breathing to return to a normal rhythm.

You will begin to feel a change come over your entire body. Gradually you will become less aware of your breathing, but not captured in your stream of consciousness. Consciousness is encouraged on the whole, but we often are too alert and hyper-stimulated via TV, caffeine, family life, just to name a few. By breathing for 5 minutes daily, you will become more centered inward. You will just live "in the moment," in your own skin.

Benefits of a simple breathing exercise throughout the day include:
- Calming
- "Re-centering" one's thoughts
- Increase in oxygenated blood flow, improved efficiency expiring carbon dioxide
- Decreased levels of fatigue later in the day, legs won't feel "heavy"

Increasing oxygenated blood via deep breathing can decrease muscle pains, especially in the postural muscles (back and neck muscles), and help counteract chronic stressors such as sitting or standing in static positions for extended periods of time.

Deep Breathing
Practice deep breathing as a form of relaxation before bed. Slow, deep breathing is an excellent way to slow the heart rate and contemplate the day's events. Focus on breathing in through the nose and out through the mouth.

Simple Stress Reliever

Looking for a simple, healthy way to help get through the day? Try breathing exercises—a wonderfully effective way to reduce stress, maintain focus, and feel energized. Exhaling completely is one breathing exercise to try—it can promote deeper breathing and better health.

Give it a try: Simply take a deep breath, let it out effortlessly, and then squeeze out a little more. Doing this regularly will help build up the muscles between your ribs, and your exhalations will soon become deeper and longer. Start by practicing this exhalation exercise consciously, and before long it will become a healthy, unconscious habit.

CHAPTER FIVE

Path to Better Health:

Benefits of Exercise

Exercise for a Healthy Brain

Along with proper diet and adequate amounts of sleep, exercise can be very effective in improving brain health by helping to create new neurons. As a caregiver that is overseeing the day-to-day care of a client with dementia, it's vital to understand how exercise effects brain health.

How is this possible? Neurons primarily grow in the hippocampus (see illustration) through a process called neurogenesis. If the hippocampus is starved of oxygen (a condition called hypoxia) it can hinder learning and memory capacity and, if left untreated, it may result in conditions such as Alzheimer's. Exercise aids in neurogenesis by increasing blood flow to the brain and stimulating the nervous system through new and challenging exercise movements.

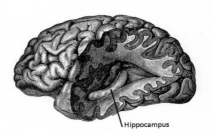

Hippocampus

Learning complex exercises and movements like the ones in this book is a proven way to strengthen the brain. Building a buff brain and building a buff body are both realistic goals, as long as one commits oneself to challenging the mind and body.

What Type of Exercise is Best for Dementia Patients?

Learning exercises that require thought, rather than mindless repetition, is vitally important because more neurons are grown during tasks that require extensive mental effort to both learn and master. To increase the difficulty of exercises, we can adjust several variables including reps, sets, weight, time under tension, and range of movement. The Programs in Chapter 8 are specifically designed to continue challenging the brain while also strengthening the body.

While physical activity (such as the exercises in this book) and cognitive engagement (for example, playing the piano) are not the only ways to prevent neural degeneration, they may delay the on-set of dementia and can also alleviate signs or symptoms of such conditions.

Remember:
Be sure to practice the Techniques on pages 66-68 with your patient or loved one every day to improve brain health!

The hippocampus is one of the centers for memories, learning, and emotion, which explains why research has found that the hippocampus shrinks in even mild cases of Alzheimer's, causing the various emotion- and memory-related symptoms described in Chapters 2 and 3. This is why stimulating all of the senses through physical, social, and cerebral activities are significant steps in reducing the severity of brain damage. Examples include physical activity, participating in a local choir group, or working on a crossword puzzle. Early intervention with these types of activities can assist in slowing down the degenerative process of the brain by stimulating the emotional, learning, and memory centers of the brain

The most important point to note is that new nerve cells form every single day in the brain, but if we don't use them, we'll lose them. This same principle applies to our muscles: if we don't exercise regularly, our muscles will atrophy, shrink, and lose size. To prevent this from happening in the brain, make sure to play new brain games every few days.

Fun brain games include:
- Sudoku
- Trivia games
- Crossword puzzles
- Board games
- Jigsaw puzzles

Exercising with Arthritis or Other Restrictions

What are your options for exercise if your loved one already has arthritis, joint pain, or restrictions in movements such as walking or getting up and down out of a chair? The answer is to first identify the activities that cause pain or soreness and then develop a realistic strategy to address the stressors that are causing the ailments (for example, if you enjoy playing tennis but you experience soreness in your knees each time you play, you may consider strengthening the areas above and below the knee through stretching and remaining flexible in your hips and ankles to alleviate stress on your joints).

The Importance of Consistency

The exercise programs in this book should become a routine in a dementia patient's daily activities due to their tendency to become easily confused. Establishing a regimen is important because changes in the program can cause confusion and may result in emotional shifts. The emotional shift may require the termination of the exercise session. You should talk clearly and directly to the person if this becomes the case.

Physical Benefits from Exercise

Improving Flow of Oxygen, Blood, and Nutrients to the Brain

By incorporating exercise into a daily routine, dementia patients can improve their heart rate, which ultimately helps the flow of oxygen, blood, and nutrients to the brain and aids in overall function of this vital organ.

Research from the University of North Carolina has shown that cerebral blood flow is increased and age-related brain alterations can be reduced with regular exercise. Active vs. Sendentary participants were compared. Active participants showed a larger amount of small blood vessels and blood flow in the brain, thus increasing oxygen delivering to brain tissue.

Increasing Flexibility and Releasing Tight Muscles

For those suffering from conditions including Alzheimer's, Vascular Dementia, and Parkinson's, the benefits of stretching are numerous.

Static stretching involves holding the muscles for 30-45 seconds. While this is great for relaxing and increasing general flexibility, new research indicates that static stretching decreases responsiveness in the nervous system, which can increase the likelihood of falls for dementia patients.

On the other hand, active stretching involves pulling back on the muscles for 5 seconds, releasing, pulling back for another 5 seconds, and then releasing again. This type of stretching activates the nervous system more than static stretching, so it is important to have a combination of both static and active stretching. Static stretching relaxes the muscles, and then active stretching opens the muscles and activates the nervous system. I recommend performing active stretching before exercise and then using static stretching after exercise. Think of active stretching as 'tricking' the muscle to relax by shutting down its natural protective mechanism, called the myotactic reflex.

The types of flexibility exercises included in an exercise program for dementia should involve a foam roller, isometrics that contract and relax the muscles, and balance training for fall prevention. The Programs in this book combine static and active stretching at the right times, along with the proper arm-up before exercising, to establish a safe and effective routine.

Improved Posture

Postural instability is the inability to maintain upright posture in standing positions and during movements. Exercise improves posture by strengthening the muscles in the spine and increasing body awareness and coordination, resulting in more efficient movement and stability with less effort.

A Note on Posture

An important aspect of improving posture is to gain awareness of the shoulders, middle back, and lower back. Have your patient or loved one begin on all fours, as shown below. Then, help them to identify these areas by first sliding the shoulder blades back and forth, arching the middle back up and down, and finally rolling the hips back and forth.

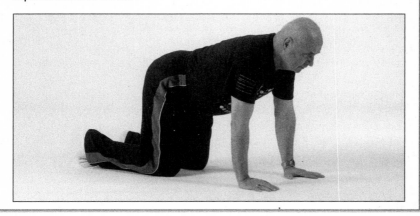

Reflexes

The threat of falling is a constant worry for those with dementia, and also persons with brittle bone diseases such as osteoporosis. Slowed reflexes are often to blame for frequent falls because our muscle fibers lose strength as we age due to hormones and lack of use, making it harder for our bodies to respond to reflexes. Balance training, partner exercises, and catching balls are all exercises that can help improve reflexes.

Pain Reduction

Exercise enhances mood by stimulating the release of endorphins. This acts as a natural pain medication, and explains why people generally feel better after 30-45 minutes of physical activity. For example, the hormone dopamine (which acts as the body's natural pain reliever) is in short supply in Parkinson's patients. But exercising stimulates dopamine production, thus deterring or delaying the side effects of Parkinson's.

Down to the Core: Training the Mid-Section

Studies show that 90% of the population experiences spine symptoms at least once in a lifetime. Hence, training the core is not necessarily about training only the abdominals, but rather the entire unit that begins with a healthy spine and back musculature working together through proper coordination and timing.

Training the core contributes to increased performance (i.e. ease of daily activities), injury prevention (i.e. fall prevention), and less overall energy requirements (i.e. improved mobility).

As you work through the exercises in this book, pay particular attention to strengthening the abdominals, hips, and groin muscles that work together to support the back and spine. Considering the neurological implications of dementia, these muscles are of particular importance. Think of the spine as a center point that allows the big muscles to contract effectively and move together in fluid movements.

These fluid movements involve communication between the opposite sides of the body namely between the shoulders and hips. Several exercises in Chapter 7 were designed to strengthen and utilize this range of motion.

Foam Rolling

Myofascial treatment ("myo" meaning muscle and "fascia" meaning specialized connective tissue) can be performed throughout the body through a technique called foam rolling.

Foam rolling helps improve body awareness and coordination, and can decrease cellulite visibility in noticeable locations such as the thighs. Foam rolling also improves circulation and blood flow to tissues, which helps alleviate symptoms of medical conditions such as Fibromyalgia.

Foam rolling addresses body systems/functions affected directly or indirectly by dementia:

- Nervous System
- Muscular System
- Joints
- Circulatory System
- Connective Tissue

Benefits of foam rolling for those with dementia include:
- Calming of the nervous system, which tends to be overactive in Parkinson's
- Release of trigger points in muscles
- Improved mobility in joints
- Decreased edema (accumulation of swelling beneath the skin) and peripheral swelling in limbs and lymph
- Hydration of stiff connective tissues

As previously discussed, the fascia system is an interweaving system of connective tissue wrapping around every portion of our body. Hence, when this support structure is tight or dehydrated (which happens when we age—imagine a dry leaf shriveling up), our joints get tight, muscles don't contract as efficiently, and we generally just don't move well.

When our fascia system becomes tighter and less mobile, our body awareness can decrease. Body awareness is simply sensing how your body interacts within the space around it (car driving by, stepping off a curb) and reacting appropriately. We foam roll because it re-hydrates, gets rid of muscle knots, and creates a greater sense of body awareness.

Suggested Program

As a caregiver or loved one with dementia, you can start them on a foam rolling program 3-4 times per week at 5 minutes per day. Keep in mind that it will be normal for them to feel a little bit of initial discomfort. Once you find a point on their body that is painful, hold the pressure for 45 seconds. The pain they feel in one specific area is likely a muscle knot. If the knot does not release, move away from the point slowly until the pain decreases.

When rolling, it will be important to gauge their pain response during the movements. Use a scale of 1-5 (1 being the least pain and 5 being the most pain). Over the course of several weeks, the pain responses should become less and less during your daily routine.

Visit Sue Hitzmann's website (www.meltmethod.com) for more information on foam rolling therapy.

Cognitive Benefits from Exercise

As was explained earlier, exercise leads to the release of certain neurotransmitters in the brain that have been shown to ease pain, both physically and mentally. Aerobic exercise creates connections between nerves (neurons). These connections enhance the speed and depth of how information is processed and retained.

We know that effective brain function uses a combination of mental processes that includes intuition, judgment, language and remembering.

In the Programs from Chapter 8, teach someone with Alzheimer's to use all of these elements:

Intuition: does this exercise feel right?

Judgment: what workout should I do today based upon my goals?

Language: is communicating my health goals clearly linked to my overall success?

Remembering: is this how I performed this exercise the last time I did it?

Thinking More Clearly

Increased blood flow, oxygen delivery, and endorphins are all released during exercise, resulting in greater clarity of the mind. Imagine what this increased clarity could do for someone with dementia. The benefits could include anything from remembering medications or an appointment at the doctor's office, to heightened responsive reflexes that may prevent falling.

Memory is the process of events by which we can recall learned experiences or skills for utilization, for example operating a motor vehicle. Memory is broken down into three categories: immediate, short-term, and long-term.

Dr. Anthony Goodman, M.D. describes each of these memory categorizations as the following:

Immediate Memory: Recalled in the current moment. These are things we are only aware of during the action itself, for example tapping fingers, doodling, etc.

Short-Term Memory: Recalled for a few seconds to a few minutes. All memory starts off short-term, but repetitive movements can facilitate a transfer of these memories to long-term memories.

Long-Term Memory: Learned over time. 1 percent of our total conscious information intake is long-term memory.

Increased Learning Ability

Performing exercises over and over again in the same way is encouraged in the beginning of an exercise program because it helps a dementia patient to build his or her skills. However, when he or she become increasingly confident in their physical abilities, it is important that they continue challenging themselves by changing the exercises. Here's why:

Plasticity: Ability to change learned behavior when responding to new stimuli. This ability is linked to neurogenesis, the stimulation of new neurons.

Learning: Ability to acquire new information by experience or instruction. Constantly stimulating the brain to adapt and adjust.

Social and Family Benefits from Exercise

One unique aspect of exercise is that it can be done by the patient, or with others. For those with dementia, social interaction with others is of vital importance and exercise provides this opportunity.

Group fitness classes that focus on balance, strengthening, and partner training are beneficial for dementia patients. Building stronger relationships, meeting new people, and sharing a common sense of purpose results from participating in group fitness classes.

In addition to meeting new people, exercise may provide a bridge to strengthening connections with family and friends. Because dementia can be a long and very disturbing event in the family structure, positive experiences (such as shared exercise) for the patient and their family are always welcomed.

Whether it's taking a leisurely walk with family, playing bocce ball, or a fun game of musical chairs, movement and interaction are paramount.

CHAPTER SIX

Rules of the Road:

Exercise Precautions

One of the greatest detriments to someone with dementia is fear. Particularly with Alzheimer's, dementia patients have a tendency to fall three times more often than people without cognitive impairment and the more they fall, the greater their fear of independence becomes. In the following chapter, you will find many great exercises that satisfy dementia patients' need for exercise, particularly through balance, strength, and movement-based exercises. The exercises and Programs found in Chapters 7 and 8 are specially designed to be safe and effective, even for elderly dementia patients.

Patients following the programs in Chapter 8 should not hesitate to cater the program to their own specific needs and abilities by panning through and finding the exercises they really enjoy. These are the exercises they will be more likely to perform with increased regularity and consistency, which are two key factors for achieving a healthier brain through exercise.

Through performing these exercises, they will be participating in something called "Motor Learning." It is important to keep in mind that there will be a learning curve for new physical and mental exercises, which may cause some frustration for dementia patients as they become accustomed to the movements and activities. See "Maintaining Motivation" on page 49 for tips on keeping the patient motivated and preventing frustration throughout the learning process.

The first few weeks of the Program is called the cognitive (verbal) stage, during which they will be mentally figuring out what to do. This should last 3-4 weeks.

During the second learning stage, named the associative stage, they should be able to perform the action, but possibly with errors. This should last 2-3 weeks.

Lastly, the automatic stage is when they are able to perform the exercises without error (or, with "great form") and can repeat sets and reps week after week.

Exercise Categories

This book's exercise program is broken down into three primary categories:
1. **Stability**
2. **Stamina**
3. **Movement**

Stability

Stability training teaches the body to stabilize the hips, back, and shoulders. We then apply strength exercises like squats or lunges, called resistance training.

Core Stability

Core training has gotten a lot of press since the mid-nineties, when greater awareness its importance began to become common knowledge. The result of core training, core strength, could more appropriately be called core stability.

Forward bending and backward extensions occur in what is called a sagittal plane of motion. Examples of common exercises that occur in this plane are toe touches and back extensions, both of which are dynamic movements.

Stamina

Stamina focuses on building the energy systems of the body, and involves maintaining energy and strength for a long period of time while performing a particular activity. The exercises in this book work on building one's

Planes of the Body

Sagittal Plane (Lateral Plane)

A vertical plane running from front to back; divides the body or any of its parts into right and left sides.

Coronal Plane (Frontal Plane)

A vertical plane running from side to side; divides the body or any of its parts into anterior and posterior portions.

Transverse Plane (Axial Plane)

A horizontal plane; divides the body or any of its parts into upper and lower parts.

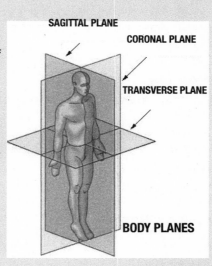

total work capacity (functional capacity) by changing rest intervals, and incorporating circuits and functional exercises such as walking up and down stairs or picking up objects.

Developing endurance or stamina and work capacity are two primary goals of *Exercises for Brain Health*. Endurance is broken down into two types, cardio-respiratory and muscular. These are defined by the Centers for Disease Control as follows:

Cardio-respiratory Endurance
Cardio-respiratory endurance is the ability of the body's circulatory and respiratory systems to supply fuel during sustained physical activity (USDHHS,1996 as adapted from Corbin & Lindsey, 1994). To improve the cardio-respiratory endurance, have the Alzheimer's patient try activities that keep his or her heart rate elevated at a safe level for a sustained length of time such as walking, swimming, or bicycling. The chosen activity does not have to be strenuous to improve cardio-respiratory endurance. Have them start slowly with an activity they enjoy, and gradually work up to a more intense pace.

Muscular Endurance

Muscular endurance is the ability of the muscle to continue to perform without fatigue (USDHHS, 1996 as adapted from Wilmore & Costill, 1994). To help someone improve his or her muscular endurance, have them try cardio-respiratory activities such as walking, jogging, bicycling, or dancing.

Movement

Movement consists of flexibility training, soft tissue rolling, and balance training.

The movement section of exercises focuses on increasing body temperature, improving body awareness, enhancing coordination, and self-applied soft tissue therapy. A recent *New York Times* article entitled "Stretching: The Truth" discusses the benefits of movement-based exercises for increasing overall functional capabilities.

The article notes, "A well-designed warm-up starts by increasing body heat and blood flow. Warm muscles and dilated blood vessels pull oxygen from the bloodstream more efficiently and use stored muscle fuel more effectively.

They also withstand loads better. One significant if gruesome study found that the leg-muscle tissue of laboratory rabbits could be stretched farther before ripping if it had been electronically stimulated—that is, warmed up."

Cognitive Strategies

One of the best ways to keep the brain sharp is to exercise. According to the Mayo Clinic, the secret to improving memory is exercise—something you already know is good for you. In fact, research has shown that exercise is a large contributor to brain power as well as aiding in the battle against Alzheimer's and aging-related memory loss.

Secondly, learning new skills, whether physical or mental, stimulates "plasticity" in the brain through the generation of new neurons (neurogenesis), ultimately helping to improve memory and language. This is why we learn!

Brain Exercises

Exercise helps with all kinds of memory, including sensory (physically remembering a motion), short-term (recalling new daily medications) and long-term (getting home).

> **Remember:**
> Be sure to practice the Techniques on pages 66-68 with your
> patient or loved one every day to improve brain health!

Strategies for memory enhancement include the following:
- Interest (engage in enjoyable pastimes)
- Note-taking (focus and review)
- Understanding (break down the parts so that you can teach it to others)
- Categorize similar concepts through visualization (create a mind-map, write something out in pictures) or mnemonics (creative ways to remember information, for example, "Every Good Boy Does Fine," can be used to remember the musical notes E, G, B, D, and F)

As we discussed in earlier chapters, just like any other muscle, the brain needs to be exercised in order to keep it strong, so it is very important to keep the mind active. Word games, puzzles and game shows are all good ways of keeping the mind working. It is good to remind those suffering from dementia that occasional, minor memory lapses are normal in individuals of all ages.

Maintaining Motivation
Having self-confidence in one's mental and physical abilities can be half the battle in preventing premature mental decline. Here are suggestions that will help dementia patients, but sources such as the Mayo Clinic or the Cleveland Clinic may have additional helpful information tailored to your needs. See the Resources section on page 146 for information on how to contact helpful organizations.

- **Believe in yourself:** When exposed to negative stereotypes about aging and memory, middle-aged and older learners tend to forget more. Yet, under the influence of messages about memory preservation into old age, performance ranks from normal to above-average.
- **Make the most of what you have:** Use calendars, planners, maps, shopping and reminder lists, file folders, and address books to keep routine information accessible. For items you use and lose frequently—keys, glasses, or change, start putting them in one place.

Brain Games: The New Age of Interactive Brain Training

Video games, computer-learning software, and hand-held devices like the Progio are examples of the newest technologies for interactive health media. Attention, memory, cognitive control and processing speed are four areas that these types of games and devices attempt to improve.

Many of us have heard of programs such as Wii Sports, Nintendo's gaming software that allows users to improve motor skills (for example, hand/eye coordination) through sporting activities such as bowling and tennis. Not only are these types of programs helpful for dementia patients living at home, but Wii Sports is also now being used for cognitive therapy in nursing homes because it emphasizes focus, motor learning, and response to stimuli (for example balance training) In fact, Medicare is now getting on board by funding experimental brain games in nursing homes and assisted living centers.

There are also several other memory-improvement courses that are becoming available. Consult with the patient's neurologist, therapist, or aging specialist on the specific benefits of a program you are interested in pursuing. Focus on courses that address real-life activities that may include scheduling appointments, word association games, or simple foreign language courses that they can try out in your local community.

- **Help yourself:** If you can, break information into smaller chunks. It's easier to remember parts of a phone number than numbers for your entire family. Or consider how it was always easier when you were in school to learn first names of individuals rather than everyone in the class at once.
- **Use your senses:** Scent is, surprisingly, the strongest sense. The oddest scents can bring back memories of childhood, friends, new cars or cooking with Mom faster than talking about it. Or consider how singing has been proven to help memory when studying—all your senses can provide surprising grounds for important memories.
- **Challenge your brain:** Reading aloud, drawing a picture, or writing down the information you want to learn widens areas in your brain involved with learning by altering tradition and expecting increased performance and involvement. Forming visual images makes it easier to remember and understand; it forces your brain to reinterpret the original information to make it more precise.

- **Repeat: Remembering new information can be as simple as repeating it out loud.** For example, if you've just met someone, say their name again when you speak with him or her: "So, Fred, how do you know my friend Tammy?"
- **Make a mnemonic:** Mnemonics can take the form of acronyms to help you remember lists. A classic example of a mnemonic is "My Very Eager Mother Just Served Us Nine Pizzas" to remember the order of the planets: Mercury, Venus, Earth, Mars, Jupiter, Saturn, Uranus and Pluto.

The Caregivers' Exercise Essentials Checklist

Exercise Preparation
- **Exercise Location:** Is your environment safe, clean, and free of debris?
- **Proper Footwear:** Are you wearing proper athletic footwear?
- **Comfortable Athletic Wear:** Do you have clothes that allow freedom of movement?
- **Hydration:** Be sure to drink 6 glasses of fluid over the course of your day.
- **Assistive Devices:** Wall mounted rails, sturdy handrails on the stairs, etc.

Exercise Equipment
- **Rolled-up towel:** can be used for resistance training, balancing on the floor, etc.
- **Mirror:** provides visual feedback on cueing and technique
- **Dumbbells:** 5-10 lb range is generally appropriate
- **Therabands:** light colored bands offer less resistance and dark colored bands offer more resistance
- **Physio-ball:** inflate the ball to the point where you can press your thumb on the surface without it sinking in
- **Tennis ball or racquet ball:** for hand and foot therapy

Playing it Safe: Important Safety Precautions

Body Positioning: Have the patient brace the core, achieve proper alignment, feel the placement of their feet, and always move first from their core before moving their limbs.

Have Them Keep a Brain Health Journal: In this journal, they can record how they're feeling on any given day and what activities they did during that time. The patient should also record what kinds of exercises they did on

51

each day and how they felt during and after their exercise session. Keeping track of this information will help both you and your loved one to better understand their health.

Rate of Perceived Exertion (RPE): You can use provide the chart below to help someone with Alzheimer's gauge how hard they are working during their session.

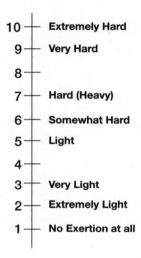

Talk Test: This is another useful way for someone to determine how hard they're working. As a person is exercising, they can gauge how easily they are able to converse and use the guidelines below to figure out the intensity of the exertion.

If they can carry on a normal conversation while exercising, they are likely working aerobically, which means the body is using oxygen as its primary energy source. If someone can work aerobically for up to 30-45 minutes, their body will also be using fat as an energy source, which is an excellent foundation for building your exercise program.

Anaerobic work, characterized below as medium intensity, should be introduced 8 weeks into an exercise program. Examples include hill walking, bike sprints, etc. When performing anaerobic exercise, they may notice their leg muscles starting to feel a bit tight, their chest will expand, they will begin to sweat, and their heart rate will reach about 40-50 beats above their resting heart rate (see below for more details on determining your heart rate).

- **Low Intensity:** Complete sentences, breathing rate normal
- **Medium Intensity:** Broken sentences, breathing rate slightly labored
- **High Intensity:** Cannot converse, breathing rate labored

Be sure someone suffering from Alzheimer's visits their healthcare provider regularly for check-ups.

Blood Pressure: This can be measured by a doctor using an electronic or manual cuff.

Determining Heart Rate: To determine someone's heart rate, place the tips of your index, second and third fingers on their wrist, below the base of their thumb. You can also place the tips of your index and second fingers on their neck, along either side of your windpipe. During exercise, it is recommended that the pulse is found on the wrist, rather than on the neck.

While pressing lightly with your fingers, you should be able to feel someone's pulse. If you don't feel their pulse, move your fingers around slightly until you find it.

Watch the second hand of a clock or watch and count the number of beats you feel in 10 seconds. Using that number, you can calculate someone's heart rate with the formula below:

$$(\text{Beats in ten seconds}) \times 6 = (\text{Heart Rate})$$

Adults over 18 years of age typically have a resting heart rate of 60-100 beats per minute. To better understand a person's heart rate, you should check their pulse before, and immediately after, they exercise. This will give you a better idea of what their body normally does at rest, and to what level their heart should be working during an exercise session.

Calculating Target Heart Rate

Your target heart rate is the level of exertion you should aim for when exercising in order to gain the most benefits from your workout. Your target heart rate is also a useful range for how your body is responding to your workout.

Target heart rate is 60-80% of your maximum heart rate, depending on what level of exertion you wish to work at.

Different Training Zones

Below is a list of the different levels of exertion and the corresponding percentage you would use to target heart rate:

Recovery Zone - 60% to 70%

Active recovery training should fall into this zone (ideally at the lower end). It's also useful for very early pre-season and closed season cross training when the body needs to recover and replenish.

Aerobic Zone - 70% to 80%

Exercising in this zone will help to develop your aerobic system and, in particular, your ability to transport and utilize oxygen. Continuous or rhythmic endurance training, like running and hiking, should fall under this heart rate zone.

Anaerobic Zone – 80% to 90%

Training in this zone will help to improve your body's ability to deal with lactic acid. It may also help to increase your lactate threshold. To determine your target heart rate, you can use the formulas below to calculate your maximum heart rate, and to then find your target heart rate.

220 – age = maximum heart rate

Maximum heart rate x training % = target heart rate

For example, if a 50 year old woman wishes to train at 70% of her maximum heart rate, she would use the below calculations:

220 – 50 = 170

170 x 70% = 119

She would thus aim to reach a heart rate of 117 during her exercise in order to work at her target heart rate.

You can also use the Karvonen Formula, which is based on both maximum heart rate and resting heart. Visit *www.sport-fitness-advisor.com/heart-rate-reserve.html* for more information.

Important Assessments

Medical Tests: Medical tests include blood panels, neurological/reflexive tests, updated family history, stress test, etc. These are tests that someone's medical provider can provide based upon his/her clinical assessment of health and risk profile. Encourage an Alzheimer's patient to have an open dialogue with his or her medical practitioner, particularly if he or she has a history of heart problems.

Six Minute Walking Test: This test is best done on a track as this will make it easier for you to judge the distance your client or loved one has covered in the 6 minutes.

Following slightly behind the person you're caring for, have them walk for six minutes as fast as they comfortably can while being able to maintain a conversation. If, during the 6-minute test, he or she experiences dizziness, shortness of breath, lightheadedness, or are unable to complete a sentence, stop walking and allow him or her to recover while keeping the stopwatch going. Once they have recovered, continue walking until the 6 minutes have run out.

After the six minutes, have them sit down on a chair or bench and ask them to give you their Rate of Perceived Exertion (RPE, see page 52).

Name: _____ Date: _____

Age:_____ Height: _____ (inches)   Weight: _____ (lbs)

Resting Heart Rate (see page 53):_____

Time in Mins	Heart Rate	RPE	Notes (signs/symptoms)

Heart rate immediately after test _____

Total distance covered _____ (yards, etc.)

One Mile Walk Test

Name: _____ Gender: _____

Date of Birth: _____ Age:_____

Weight:_____ Resting Heart Rate:_____

Directions:

Have your client or loved one walk one mile as briskly as possible.

Record the time to finish the mile.

Measure their heart rate during the 15 seconds immediately after the walk.

Make sure they do not run and instruct them to maintain an even pace.

Do not allow them to speed up at the end of the course.

Results

Time: _____

Heart Rate: _____

As you go through the Programs and exercises in this book, keep in mind the following tips:

- Healthy living includes moving the body everyday—help the person you care for make it a habit.
- Decrease inflammation by improving nutrition: Encourage them to increase their Omega 3's, hydration, high fiber, and foods rich in antioxidants everyday.
- Learning new skills creates new synapses, or connections, in the nervous system and ultimately improves brain function.
- Community and social support networks such as family, caregivers, and loved ones all provide crucial assistance for the dementia patient.

CHAPTER SEVEN

The Exercises

Overhead Squat

Feel it Here Hips, Back, Shoulders

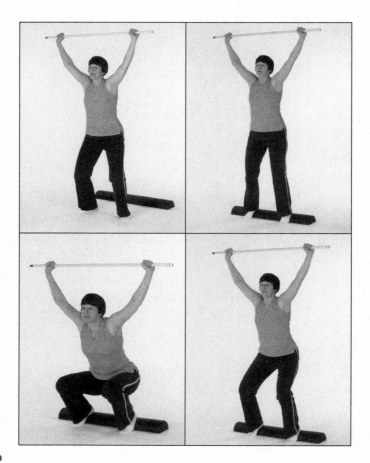

SET-UP

Position yourself with feet hip-width apart. Point your toes to 11 and 1 o'clock positions respectively, as this will allow your hips, knees, and ankles to move together properly during the squatting movement. Place the dowel (broomstick) on the crown of your head so your elbows are at a 90-degree angle, then press the stick above your head. Place a half roller under your heels if you feel your body pitching forward. Drop your hips as low as possible.

Images should be read clockwise.

Standing with Eyes Closed

Feel it Here Fully Body

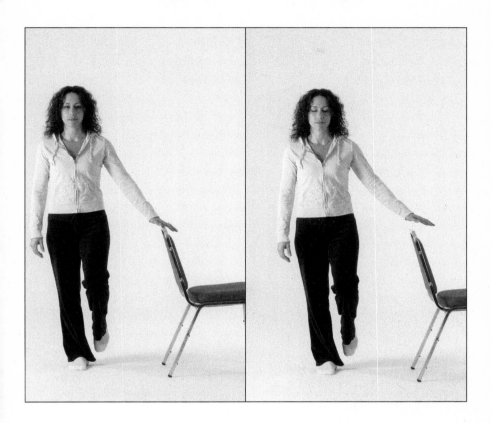

SET-UP

Stand with your feet hip-width apart. You should stand near a wall or partner for safety. For the two-legged test, rest you hands at your side and close your eyes. With both feet on the ground feel a natural sway similar to a tree in the wind. For the one-legged test, close your eyes once your foot is off the ground. With one foot on the ground the sway will increase dramatically with your body wanting to make very quick readjustments to stabilize.

Heel to Toe Walking

Feel it Here Core, Sides of Legs, Back

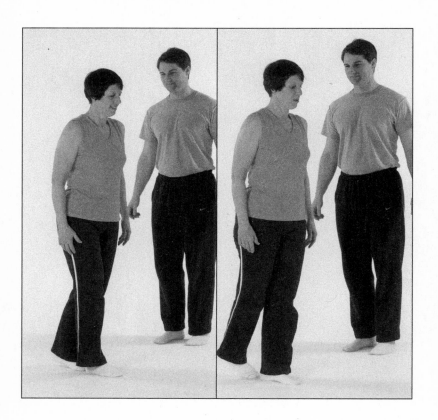

SET-UP

Find a wall or fixed surface prior to beginning this exercise in case you become off balance. Begin with your arms out to the side for added stability. Pick a spot in front of you for focus and begin the movement by placing one foot in front of the other. Experience your upper body attempting to stabilize itself more than when you are in a normal walking position. A dramatic change in stability will occur with one foot in front or behind the other. Take your time and concentrate on the placement of each foot. Repeat backwards toe-to-heel.

Getting up from a Chair

Feel it Here Core

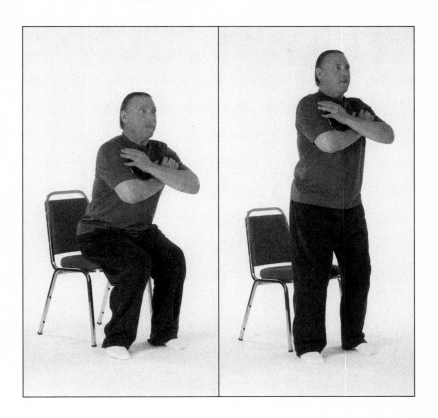

SET-UP

Position yourself on the edge of a chair. Hips should be parallel, or slightly above, knee level. Brace your core and press your feet into the ground.

Chair Sit

Feel it Here Legs

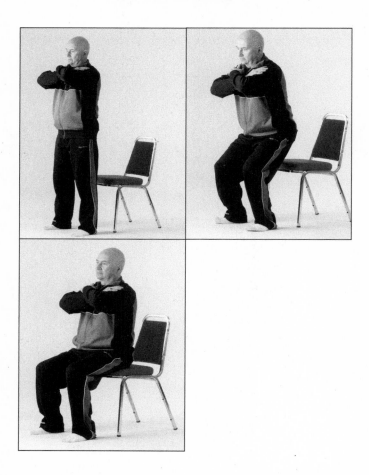

SET-UP

Using the chair as a teaching tool, lower the hips down towards the seat using legs and hips. Hold this position, relax into the chair, repeat. Work on increasing the time held for each rep. A wall can be used if the isometric squat is too much. Position your body against a wall. Walk your hips down the wall by walking your feet out in front of your body. Keep your hips, knees, and toes in line. Maintaining head, shoulder, and tailbone contact with the wall, hold the squatting position as if sitting in a chair. You should not feel pain in your knees. If you do, walk the feet out farther. Breathe into your lower body.

Push-up

Feel it Here Stomach, Chest, Arms, Legs

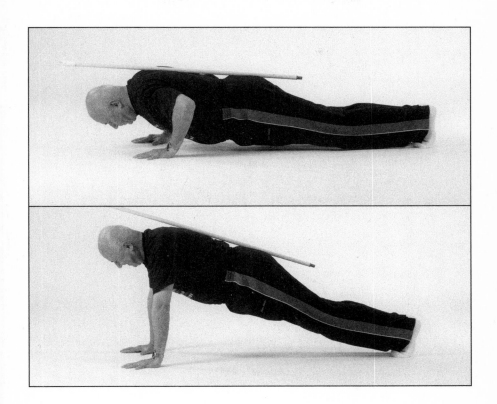

SET-UP

Position yourself on your stomach. Your hands should be parallel to your shoulders. Place a dowel stick along the spine so contact is made with your head and sacrum. Begin the movement by bracing your stomach. Push your toes and hands into the floor, then attempt to press your body away from the floor until your elbows are straight. You should feel your shoulder blades come together as you return to your starting position.

Forward Plank

Feel it Here Stomach, Legs, Shoulders

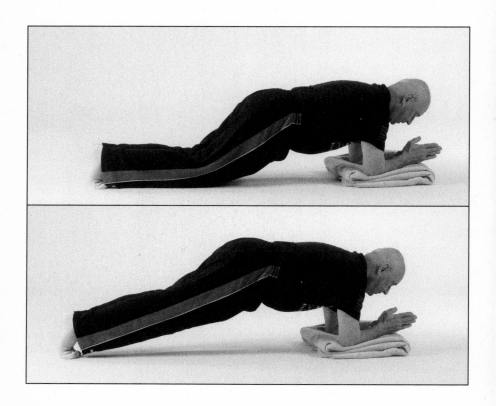

SET-UP

Position your body in the same position as a push-up, but with your hands positioned together in front of your face. To help cue the pulling of the navel to the spine, place a rolled up towel on your lower back as a bio-feedback tool. Make sure you are breathing through the entire movement. Pull your navel to the lower spine but do not flatten your lower back out. Instead, cue the lower ribs to become 'heavy'.

Lateral Plank

Feel it Here Shoulders, Ribs, Obliques, Hip

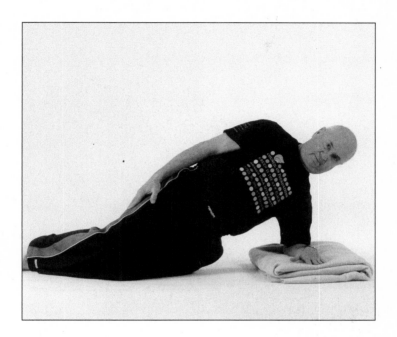

SET-UP

Position you body on one side, on your elbow and hip. Contract the side of your stomach and elevate your hip into alignment with the shoulders and knees.

Lifting Technique

Feel it Here Legs, Stomach, Spine, Shoulders, and Arms.

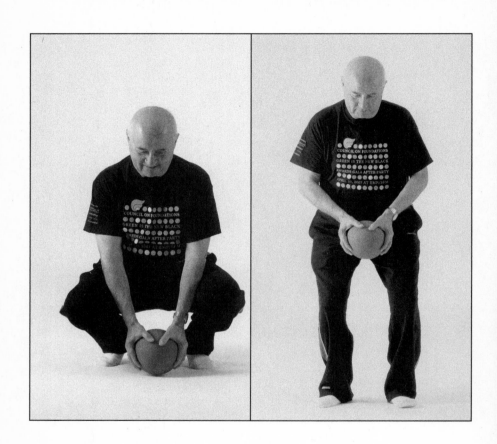

SET-UP

Point your toes to the 11 and 1 o'clock positions. Bend at the hips, knees, and ankles. Keep the object close to your body during the entire motion. Prior to beginning the upward (lifting) movement, brace your stomach and press your feet into the ground, then stand up straight. If you are unable to keep your heels down, it is especially important that you brace your stomach throughout this movement.

Rotating Technique

Feel it Here Hips, Middle Back

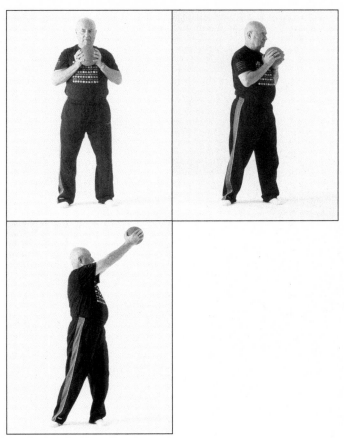

SET-UP

Set up with the same mechanics as for the lifting exercise. Keep the object as close as you can until your hips and spine reach their end points. Be careful not to twist through your lower back.

Squatting Technique
Feel it Here Legs, Back

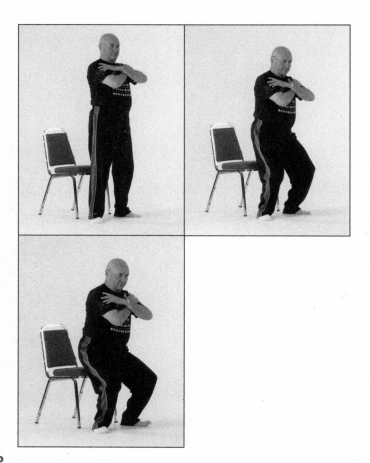

SET-UP

Cross your arms in front of your body. Hands should be resting on the front of your shoulders with elbows relaxed. Brace your stomach. Your toes should be positioned at 11 and 1 o'clock positions to allow proper movement about the hip. Look at a spot on the floor a bit in front of you, but not so much as to be entirely erect. Think about "wrinkling" your groin when squatting. This will force your hips back.

Hip Hinging

Feel it Here Lower Spine, Hamstrings,

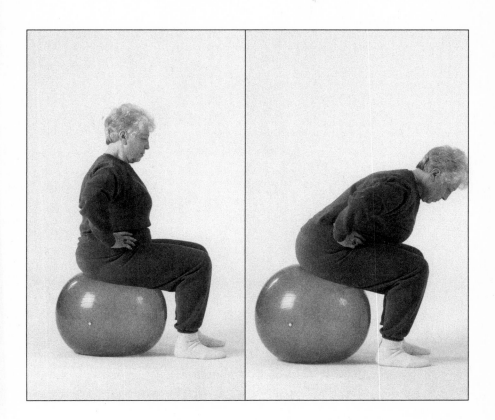

SET-UP

Start the squatting movement from your hips, letting the other parts follow. Feel your upper body positioned over the upper thighs as you bend during the downward motion. Brace your stomach, then begin the upward movement by pressing your feet into the floor, followed by pushing your hips through. For added help with stability, place a broomstick along your spine. Contact should be felt on the back of your head, middle back and tailbone.

Spinal Whip
Feel it Here Middle Back

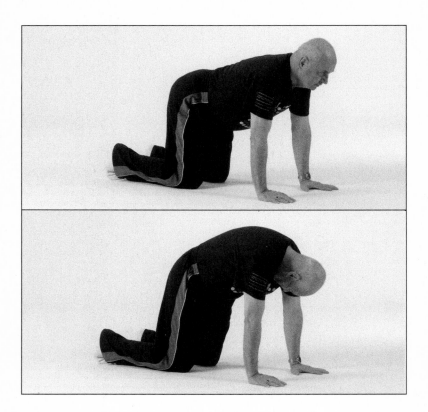

SET-UP

Begin on all fours or standing with your hands on your knees. Rotate from the shoulder blades as they move to the outside of the upper body. Emphasize moving from the middle back through the sternum.

Standing Tail Wag

Feel it Here Hips, Lower Spine

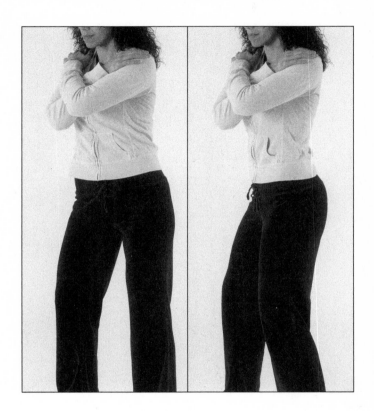

SET-UP

Square your body up facing forward. Cross your hands over your shoulders with your elbows resting on your chest. Keep your head, hips and legs quiet. Keeping your shoulders still, attempt to rotate the hips, without moving any other part of the body. Stay light through your knees.

Thoracic Flex on Roller

Feel it Here Middle Spine, Abdominals

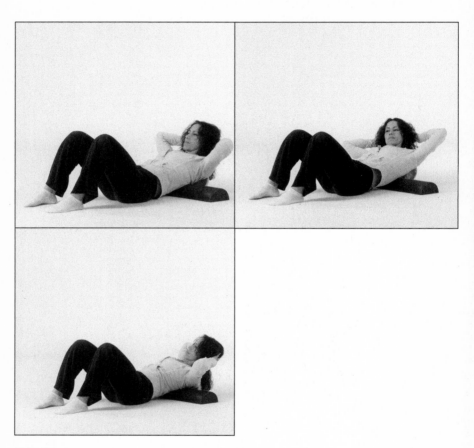

SET-UP

You can use a full roller, half roller, or thick, rolled up towel. Position the roller immediately below your shoulder blades. Your elbows should be pointed to the sides. Feel the foam roller pressing against your middle spine. Keep your ribs heavy into the ground so the core muscles are active and working through the entire motion. Your front abs will be working the entire time but the latter muscles, namely the obliques, are the actual movers.

Shoulder Circles

Feel it Here Spine

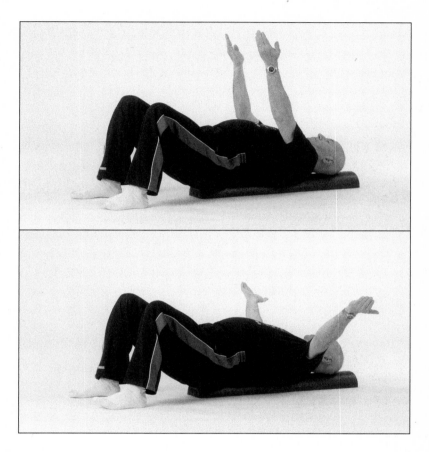

SET-UP

Lay down on the roller with your spine resting in the long position. If you need increased balance during the movement use a half roller or rolled up towel. Feel pressure on your spine. Only your head, middle back, and pelvis should be resting in contact with the roller. Initiate smooth circles with your arms as if you have a dinner tray in each hand.

Cranial Release

Feel it Here Neck

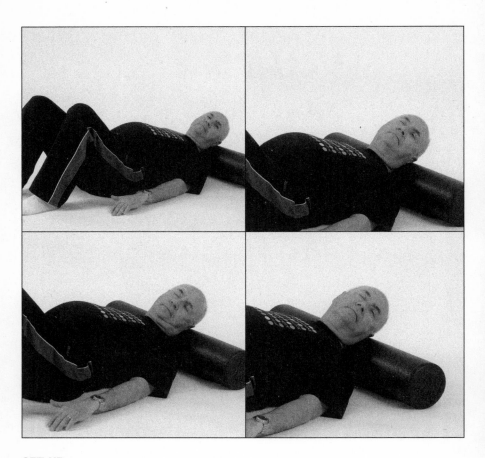

SET-UP

Lay on your back. Position the back of your head, right where it meets the base of your neck, on the roller. You should be in a comfortable position; draw your feet into your hips if needed. Your hands should be relaxed near the sides of your hips. If you need to stabilize the roller, place your hands on the sides of the roller. Rotate your head to the right and left. When rotating your head to the right and left, feel the small space that sits on either side of your head. Keep pressure in the roller by slightly extending your neck, emphasizing proper alignment. *Check out www.meltmethod.com*

Images should be read clockwise.

Sacral Release

Feel it Here Pelvis

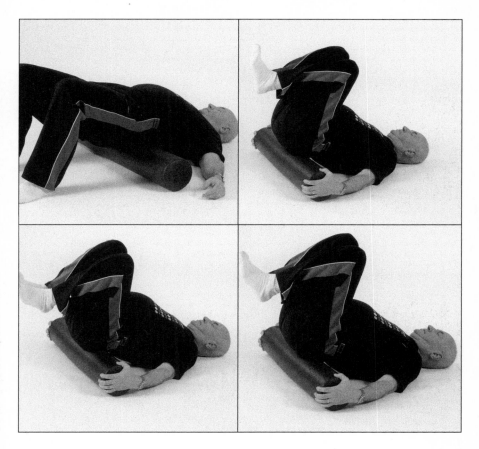

SET-UP

Position your body in a comfortable bridging position on your spine. Elevate your hips and slide the roller on your sacrum. Keeping your ribs heavy, engaging your core, pull one knee at a time up to a position over your hips. Addressing one side of your pelvis at a time, let your knees drift over until you feel a 'barrier' or place of irritability. Once found, gently make circles with your knees both ways, then switch to the other side.

Check out www.meltmethod.com

Images should be read clockwise.

75

Foam Roller Scissor Stretch

Feel it Here Core, Lower Back

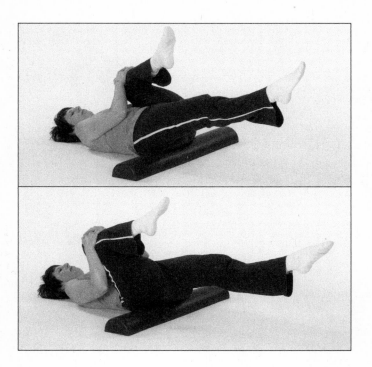

SET-UP

Lay on your back with your knees bent and feet close to your hips. Press your feet into the floor, then elevate your hips. Slide a foam roller (or very thick towel) beneath your tailbone/sacrum. Keeping your ribs heavy, pull one knee to your chest and hold. Extend the leg next, keeping ribs heavy, engaging the core. The sacrum is the flattish bone that positions itself directly below the lower back. Place the palm of your hand on the sacrum; it should fit nicely. The roller sits between the lower back and sacrum. *Check out www.meltmethod.com*

MELT Ball Series

Feel it Here Small Joints

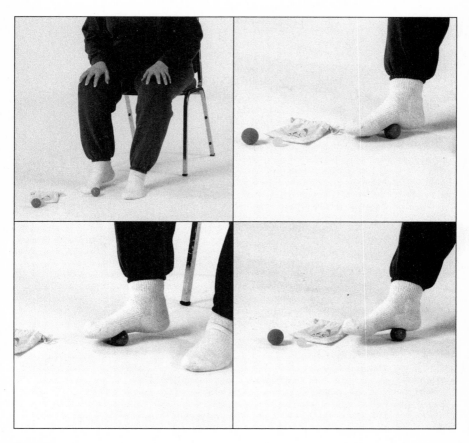

SET-UP

Apply balls to joint and soft surfaces allowing the joints/tissues to decompress and open. Compression is one of our body's enemies as we age. Similar patterns of position point pressing can be applied to the hands and feet. Do not let the balls sink into the soft tissue spaces between the joints—nerves sit there.

Images should be read clockwise.

Hip Lifters

Feel it Here Hips, Back

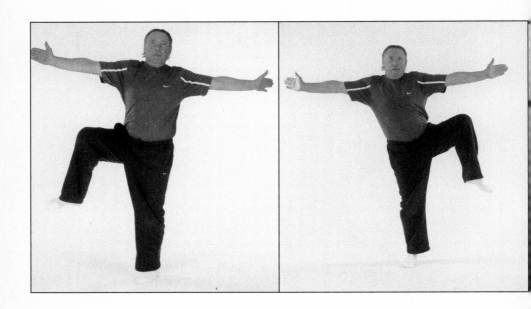

SET-UP

With hands out to the side, draw the hip out and knee up behind the arm. Feel the hips and back working throughout this exercise.

Double Arm Stretch

Feel it Here Chest, Middle & Lower Back

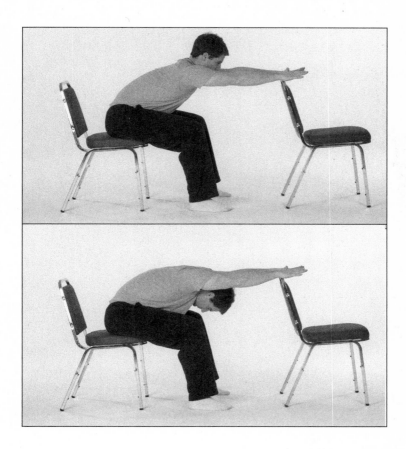

SET-UP

This stretch can be done using either a door frame or chair. For the chair stretch (see picture), use a steady chair with arms draped over. Drop your head between the arms. For the door frame, stand between a door frame that is in front of you. Place both arms up against the door frame with a 90 degree angle at the elbows. Once the arms are positioned comfortably, take a step forward, and begin to feel a stretch through your chest and shoulders.

Wrist/Forearm Stretches

Feel it Here Wrist

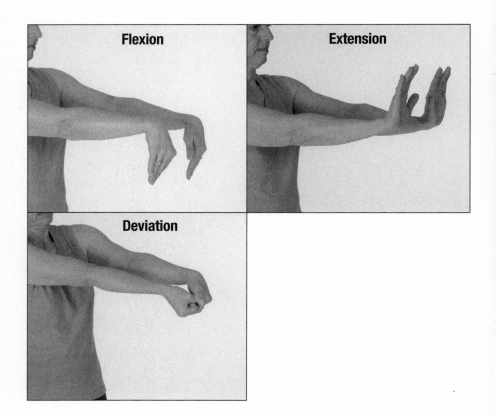

SET-UP

Flexion (Pullover): Gently provide traction to the wrist by pulling out on the hand. This will create the sensation of your hand and forearm moving away from one another. Assist the movement from the back of the middle part of the hand.

Extension (Pullback): Gently pull out on the wrist. Draw back the fingers and hand together. To intensify the stretch, pull back closer to the fingers.

Deviation (Thumb Pull): Begin by tucking the thumb into the palm of the hand. Cup the fingers of the stretching wrist around the thumb. Assist the wrist in tilting downwards while keeping the elbow straight.

Rotator Cuff Stretch

Feel it Here Shoulders

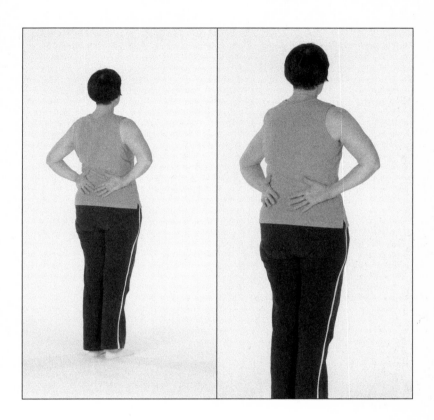

SET-UP

Shake out the shoulders. Gently press the outside of your hands into the lower back, while allowing the elbows to drift forward. Upon reaching an end point, return the elbows back to neutral and slide the hands down and out.

Double Arm Hug Rotation

Feel it Here Upper & Middle Back

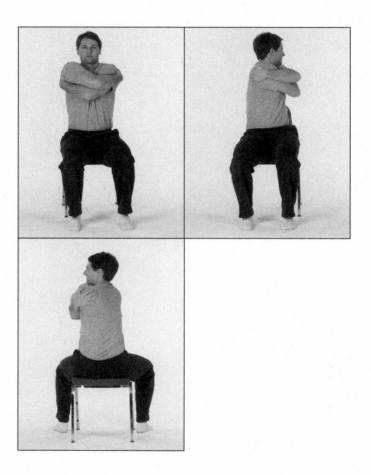

SET-UP

Sit upright on a sturdy surface. Give yourself a 'big hug'. Keeping pressure on the backs of the shoulders, rotate around your waist.

Alphabet Series: W's

Feel it Here Middle Back

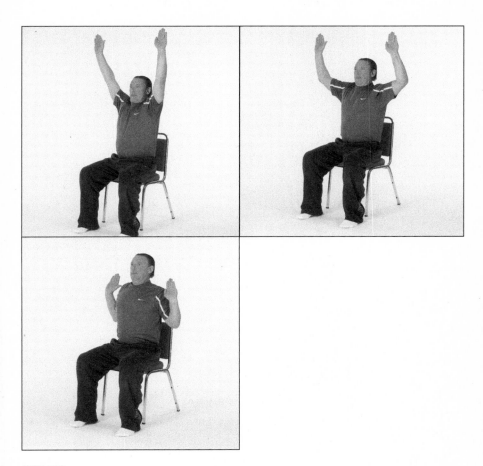

SET-UP

Sit upright on a sturdy surface. Squeeze your shoulder blades back and down. Draw both elbows down and back into the middle spine. Hold, then release.

Alphabet Series: Y's

Feel it Here Middle & Lower Back

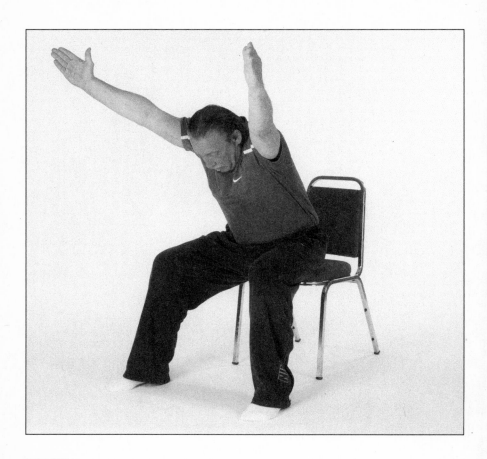

SET-UP

Sit upright on a sturdy surface. Squeeze your shoulder blades back and down. Draw both arms up, and straight out in front of your body at a 45 degree angle.

Alphabet Series: T's

Feel it Here Middle Back, Behind Shoulders

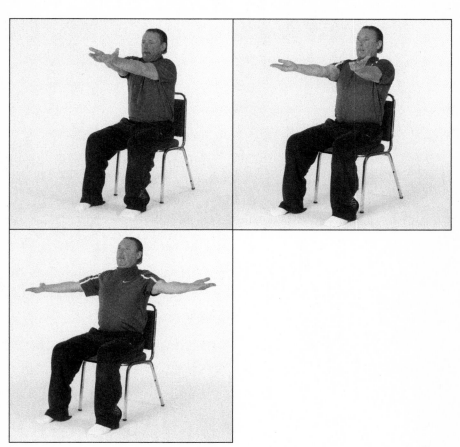

SET-UP
Sit upright on a sturdy surface. Squeeze your shoulder blades back and down. Draw both arms out from the mid-line of the body with palms up.

Ribcage Opener

Feel it Here Groin, Back, Shoulders

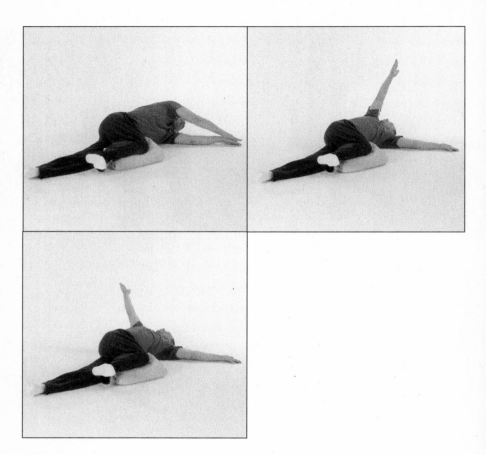

SET-UP
Lay on the ground and position a rolled up towel or foam roller under your knee. Start with your hands together. Press your knees into the object then initiate rotation with your hand. Follow the rotation down the arm until you feel it through your ribcage.

Ankle Pumps

Feel it Here Front of Shins, Calves

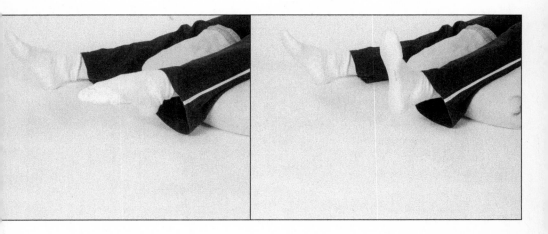

SET-UP
Gently point and flex the foot, reaching out through the front of the big toe.
Pull the toes back by pushing through the heel.

Knee to Forehead

Feel it Here Hips

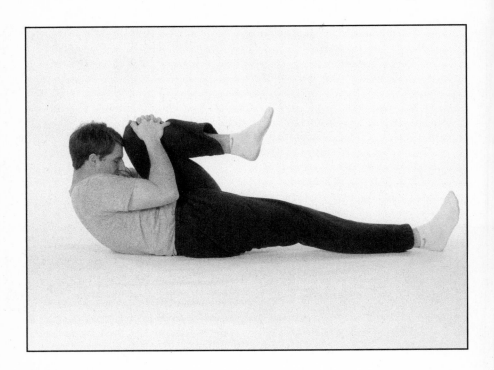

SET-UP
Tighten up the stomach. Draw the knee towards the chest, grabbing the knee with two hands.

Lateral Side Bend on Physio-ball

Feel it Here Ribcage, Shoulders, Lower Back

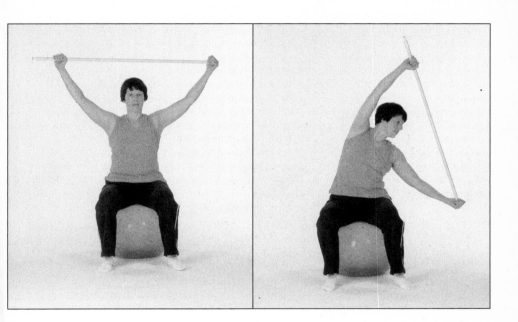

SET-UP

Sitting atop the Physio-ball, maintain a stance wider than hip-width. Push the broomstick above the head with straight arms. Initiating the motion from the hands, slowly flex the back to one side. The stick will be cupped into the bottom hand. If your opposite hip comes up, you have gone too far.

Physio-ball Roll

Feel it Here Stomach, Ribs, Chest, Shoulders

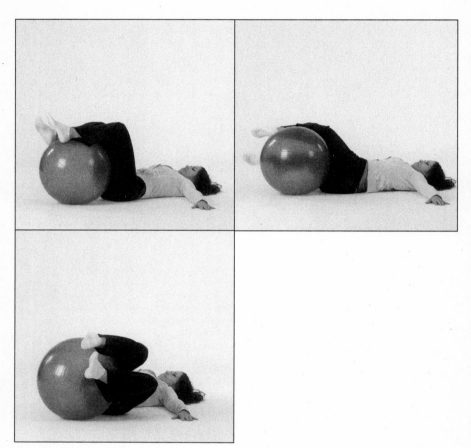

SET-UP

Cup your legs over a Physio-ball at an angle slightly greater than 90 degrees, or a square angle at the knees and hips. Position your arms out to the side with palms down to aid in stability during lower body movement. On the way toward the floor, breathe in and gently press the back of your legs into the ball thereby slowing the legs down. On the way back to your starting position, breathe out and press your hand into the floor to activate the stomach and shoulders. This stabilizes your spine prior to moving the ball.

Draw the Sword/Return the Sword

Feel it Here Back of Shoulder, Middle Back

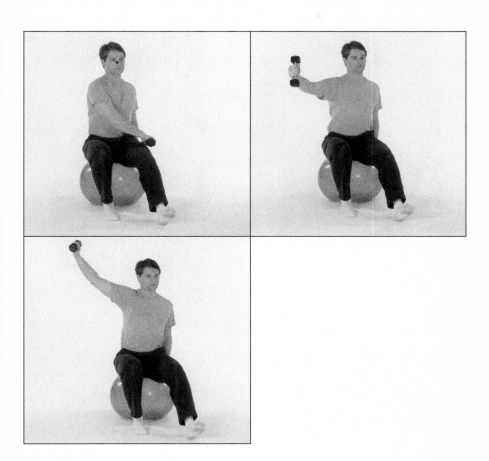

SET-UP

Imagine you are drawing a sword from the opposite side with a closed hand. Draw the sword across your body into an open hand position over the opposite shoulder. The motion is accomplished with the back muscles. The muscles run from the back of the shoulder through the middle back. Imagine your shoulder has a direct line of action drawn from the shoulder to the opposite hip. For an alternative, hold a light weight (shown above) in the hand that moves across the body.

Assisted Rotational Chair Stretch

Feel it Here Middle Back, Hips, Shoulders

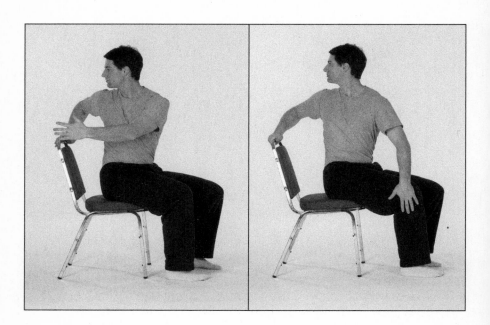

SET-UP

Begin seated with one hand on the back of the chair. Keep your feet hip-width apart. Place your other hand on your knee to use as leverage in order to achieve greater rotation. Take a deep breath in, then rotate as shown above.

Calf Raises

Feel it Here Calves, Feet

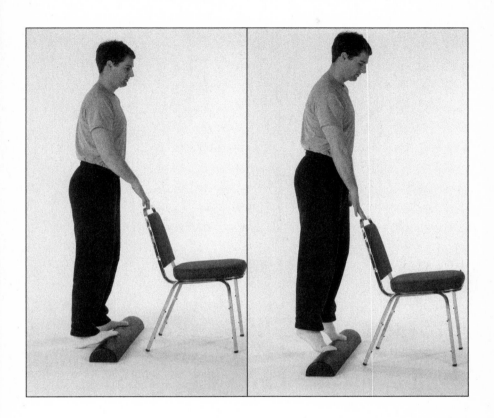

SET-UP

Stand atop a foam roller, facing a chair with your feet parallel and pointed forward. You should be able to see the front of your feet when looking down. Keep your hands light against the chair. Begin by pressing the balls of your feet into the ground, then pull your heels up towards the back of your hips. To increase the effort on the calves and feet, perform the movement higher off the ground and on a single leg.

Heel to Toe Rocks

Feel it Here Full Body

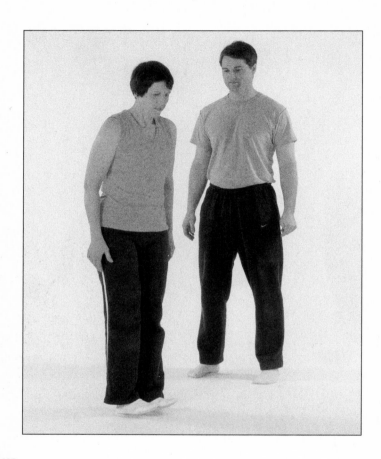

SET-UP

Partner rocks back and forth from the toes to heels as you provide support if needed.

Physio-ball Foot Lifts

Feel it Here   Hips, Legs

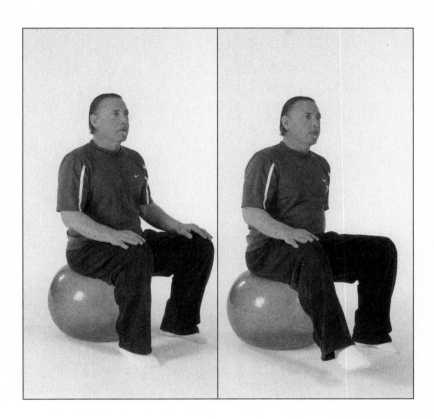

SET-UP

Sit on the very top of the Physio-ball. You should feel as if you are sitting slightly higher than on a regular chair and a bit more open in the front of the hips. Use the hip hinging cue (see page 69) to find the back alignment necessary to maintain positioning and stability. Feel braced through the core. This will stabilize your back and hips before you lift your foot. Lift one foot off the floor, hold. Work on shifting your body weight slowly to one foot prior to lifting the opposing knee/foot. Use a mirror or partner to accomplish.

Clock Series: Single Foot Touches

Feel it Here Legs, Hips

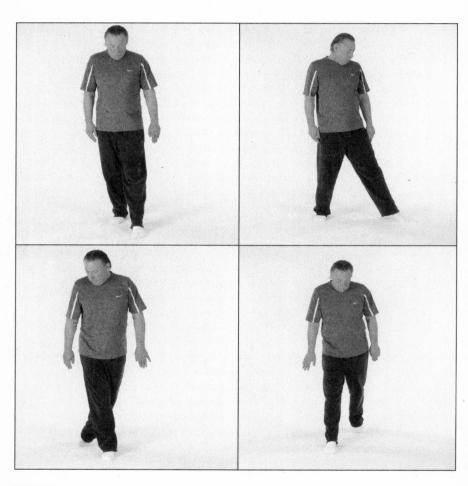

SET-UP

Imagine you are standing in the center of a clock face. Touch 2-3 numbers around the clock. As you become more comfortable, touch more numbers, then switch feet.

Images should be read clockwise.

Balancing on Half Roller

Feel it Here Hips, Quads, Calves

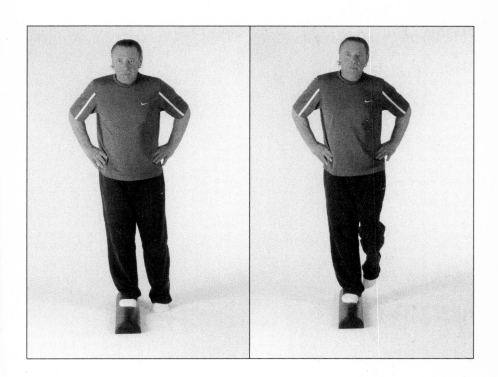

SET-UP

Step onto the roller, keeping both feet on the ground. Gently pick one foot off the ground. Expect your opposite ankle to feel unstable. Keep your core braced.

Kegel

Feel it Here Pelvic Floor, Core

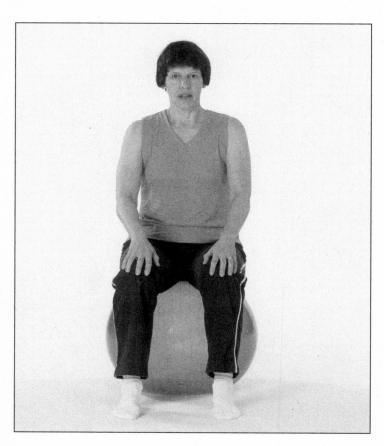

SET-UP

While keeping your lower back quiet and relaxed, squeeze your pelvic floor muscles in and up towards the pelvis. Imagine there is a balloon attached to your pelvic floor and it's rising. Try this exercise on the floor first to take surrounding muscles out of the learning curve.

All Fours Core Progression

Feel it Here Core, Middle/Lower Back

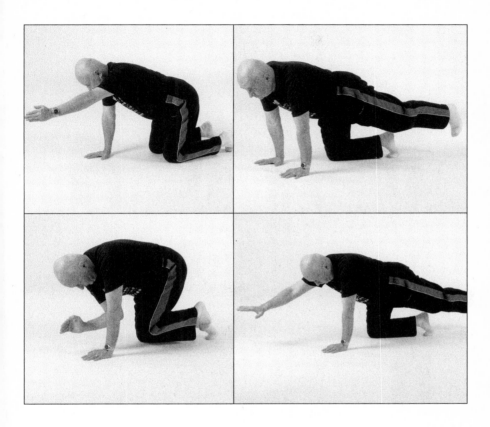

SET-UP

Begin the core series on all fours. Each progression will begin with ribs heavy and bracing the core as you draw your navel to your spine. To draw the navel in, imagine squeezing a marble in your belly button. Use a rolled up towel to keep your core active during the progressions. A small Physio-ball can be placed under your spine if you feel your back muscles are tightening up. This variation helps your body isolate movements and learn faster.

Images should be read clockwise.

Chopping Movements

Feel it Here Core, Hips

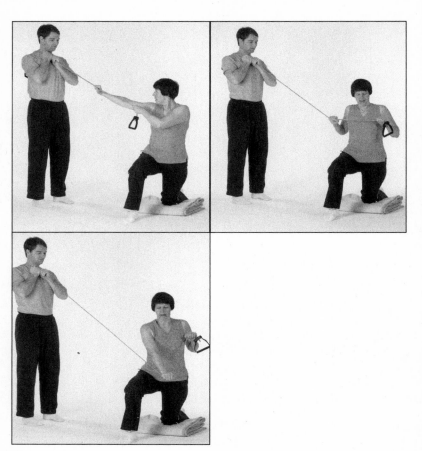

SET-UP

Chop across your body over a trailing, kneeling leg. Your front knee is on the ground on a towel or other comfortable item. Pull the band into your body, then push it down and out with the trail hand. Keep your spine neutral by concentrating on bracing your stomach and stabilizing the hips. Think about moving around a stable pillar in your spine.

Exercise provided by St. John's, AAHFRP, FMS

Lifting Movements

Feel it Here Core, Hips

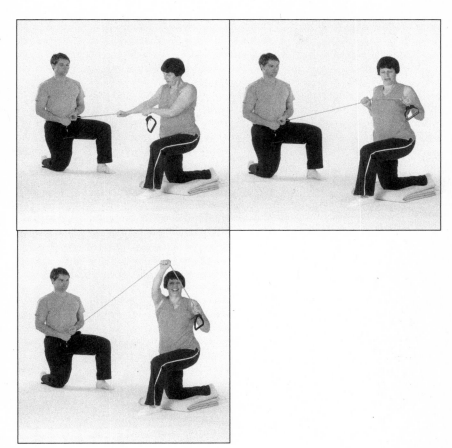

SET-UP

You will be lifting across your body over a trailing knee on the ground. The front knee should be aligned with your hip. Pull the band into your body, then push it up and out with the trailing hand. Keep your spine neutral by concentrating on bracing your stomach and stabilizing the hips. Think about moving around a stable pillar in your spine.

Exercise provided by St. John's, AAHFRP, FMS

Single Reverse Kickback on Physio-ball

Feel it Here Glutes, Lower Back

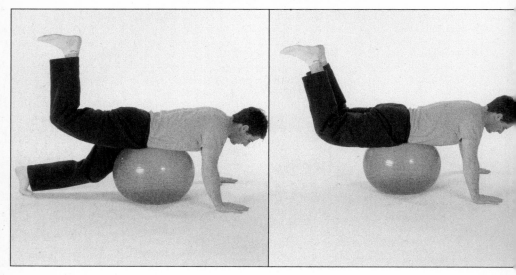

SET-UP

Start by lying face down on the Physio-ball. This exercise can be done with one leg or two legs. While maintaining balance, slowly lift one (or both) legs as shown.

Band Pulls

Feel it Here Arms, Back, Core

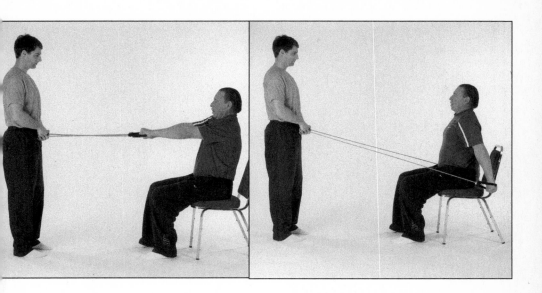

SET-UP

Keep the weight of your body in the feet and hips by slightly leaning forward. This allows the shoulders and arms to move naturally. Cue the shoulder blades to stay back and down thereby relaxing the upper neck muscles.

Band Rows

Feel it Here Back, Shoulders, Core

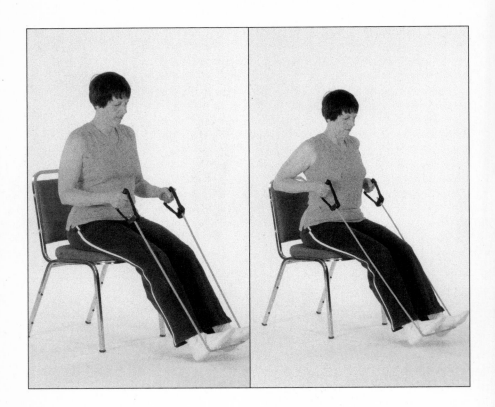

SET-UP

Position your body in an upright position on either a ball or bench. First, pull your shoulder blades back. Keeping them back, pull one elbow back at a time. Keep your ribs heavy and core contracted during each pressing repetition. Breathe out during each rep and breathe in upon return to the starting position. This exercise can also be done while standing.

Front Pullbacks

Feel it Here Core, Arms, Chest, Legs

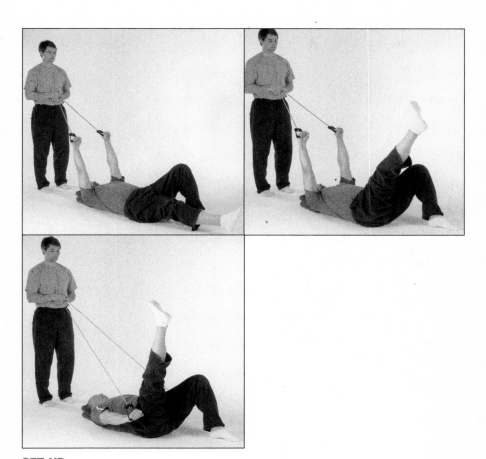

SET-UP

Begin this exercise on your back. Keeping your ribs heavy, initiate this movement from your core. Pull both arms toward one leg, pause, and return. Brace prior to each repetition.

Row with Tricep Extension

Feel it Here Back, Triceps

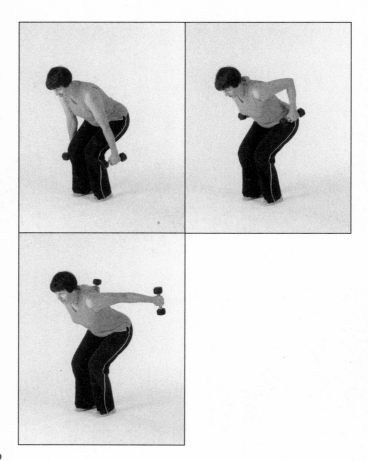

SET-UP
Either kneel (and use one arm) or stand and use both arms, shown above. Perform a row, pulling your elbows behind your back and then extend your arm fully in back of you to work the triceps.

Band Presses with Two Arms

Feel it Here Chest, Shoulders, Arms

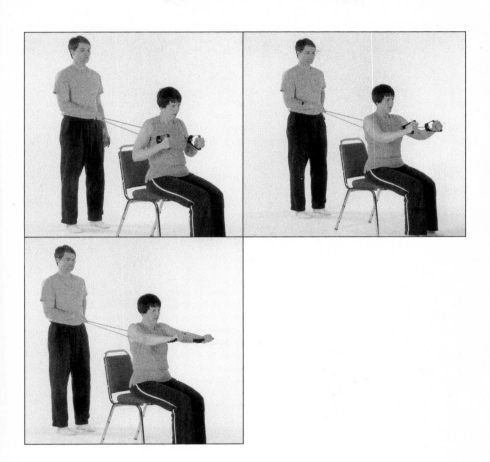

SET-UP

Position your body in a standing position in a normal stance or a split stance. Press your hands out in front until your elbows are fully extended. Keep the ribs heavy and core contracted during each pressing repetition. Breathe out during each extension and breathe in upon return to the starting position. This exercise can also be done while sitting (shown above) in an upright position on either a ball or a bench.

Band Pulls with One Knee Up

Feel it Here Core, Arms, Chest, Legs

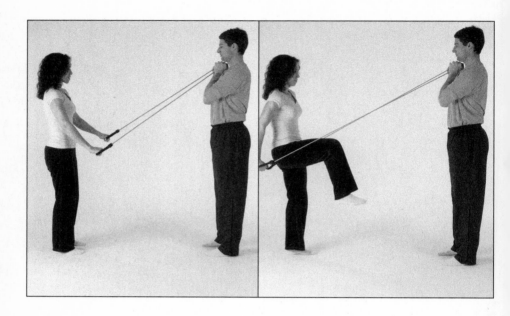

SET-UP

In a standing position, pull your knee upward towards your chest while pulling the arms to the sides of your body. Keep your ribs heavy and core contracted during each pressing repetition. Breathe out during each pressing rep and breathe out upon return to the starting position.

Towel Pulls

Feel it Here Arches and Tops of Feet, Ankles

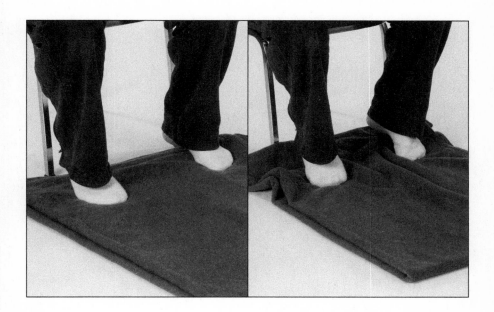

SET-UP

Take your shoes off. Lay a large towel flat on the floor. Pull the towel into the foot using the toes and arch, as shown. For added resistance, place a small weight on the towel.

Chest Stretch Open Arms

Feel it Here Chest, Shoulders

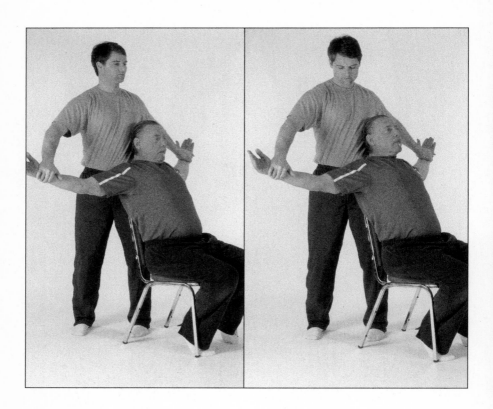

SET-UP
Stand behind your partner with your hands gently placed upon his or her upper arms. Keep your body positioned along your partner's spine to stabilize and assist in creating a greater stretch through the front of your partner's body.

110

Shoulders/Torso Stretch

Feel it Here Chest, Core, Shoulders

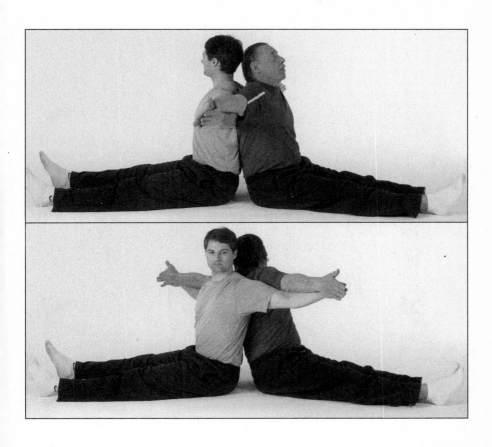

SET-UP
Sit back to back with your partner. Place palms in contact and rotate in unison.

Assisted Apley Stretch

Feel it Here Arms, Shoulders, Chest

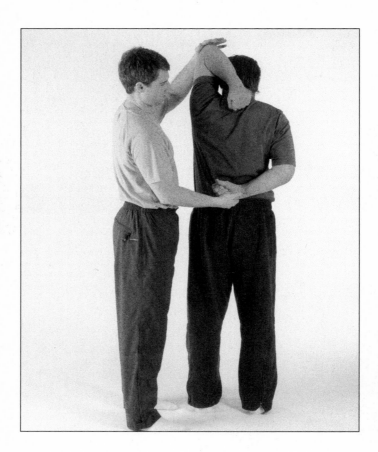

SET-UP

Instruct your partner to reach his or her arms over and under their shoulder blades, as shown above. Assist the elbows coming together while instructing your partner not to arch the middle back.

112

Double Hand Chest Press

Feel it Here Chest, Arms, Core

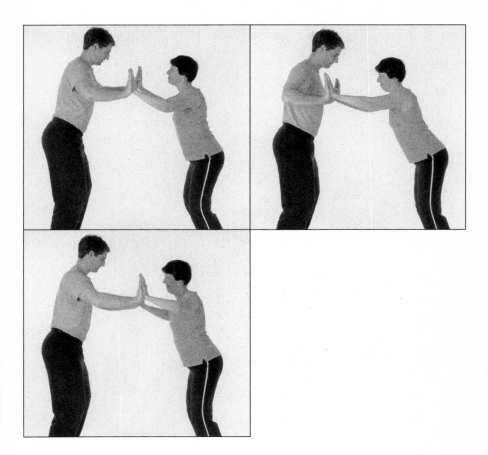

SET-UP

Press your palms against your partner's. Press your hands back and forth, resisting one another, but still allowing for range of motion similar to a dumbbell chest press. Be sure to stabilize backward through your core.

Single Hand Chest Press

Feel it Here Chest, Shoulders, Arms

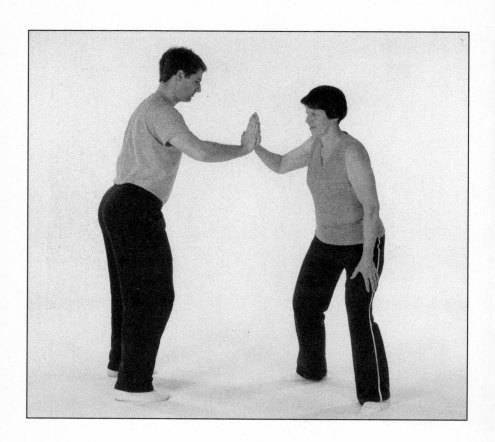

SET-UP

Using only one arm, press the palms of your hands against your partner's. Press the hands back and forth, resisting one another, but still allowing for range of motion similar to a dumbbell chest press. Be careful not to push your partner's arm too hard and be sure to stabilize forward and backward through your core.

Weight Shifting

Feel it Here Hips, Legs

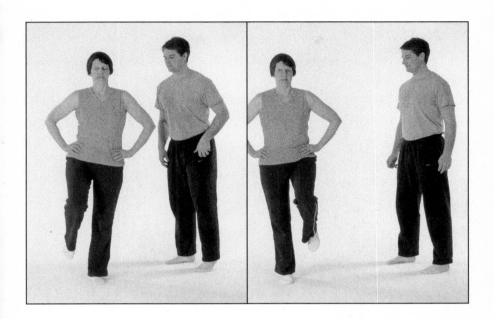

SET-UP

Your partner begins in normal walking position. As he or she walks forward, spot from the left to right leg, as your partner balances momentarily
on each leg. Partner should feel the hips and legs working to stabilize the
body during the momentary pause phase.

Partner Stability Pushes

Feel it Here Core, Spine

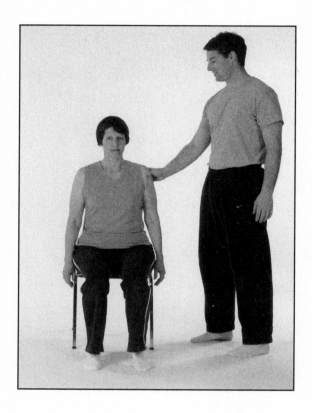

SET-UP

Partner will start in a seated position. Instruct him or her to breathe during the entire exercise. Proceed to gently push at the shoulders, middle back, and front of the body. Once your partner feels comfortable with the seated position, try the standing position. Push your partner in the same spots.

CHAPTER EIGHT

Exercise Programs and Progressions

Programs

Introductory

Cognitive
- Daily: Review daily nutrition plan (see pages 18-19 and 141)
- Weekly: Assess medications and what they are used for
- Monthly: Make 3-4 trips to the supermarket, library, or a restaurant

Physical
AM
- Start the Self-Treatment and Massage program (see page 121)
- Start the Posture program (see page 121)

Beginner

Cognitive
- Daily: Practice recalling important family members' and friends' phone numbers
- Weekly: Create and cook a series of new healthy recipes (see page 141 for ideas)
- Monthly: Plan an exercise and brain activities program in advance (see page 126 for exercise programs and pages 24, 37 and 50 for brain activities)

Physical
AM
- Start the Beginner Mobility program (see page 122)
- Start the Beginner Strength program (see page 124)

PM
- Start the Beginner Balance program (see page 123)

Intermediate

Cognitive

- Daily: Create a mnemonic of your daily, weekly, or monthly tasks (see page 51)
- Weekly: Complete a new puzzle or word game
- Monthly: Complete at least 1-2 new pieces of reading material then discuss content of the book in a small group

Physical

AM

- Start the Intermediate Strength program (see page 125) or the Stability program (see page 124)
- Start the Intermediate Balance program (see page 124)

PM

- Start the Intermediate Mobility program (see page 122)

Advanced

Cognitive

- Daily: Participate in a socially-stimulating activity such as community gardening or group discussions
- Weekly: Write out directions to medical appointments, family events, or social engagements before actually attending them
- Monthly: Plan and prepare a completely new activity using hand-eye coordination (for example, searching the Internet, using a video game, writing, or painting)

Physical

AM

- Start the Advanced Balance program (see page 123)
- Start the Advanced Strength program (see page 125)

PM

- Start the Advanced Mobility program (see page 122)

Progressions

Reps refer to the number of times you perform a movement.

A **set** represents how many times you complete a given number of repetitions of a particular exercise. Be sure to rest for a few seconds between sets.

Rest refers to the time taken between each set of exercises.

RPE refers to Rate of perceived Exertion. See page 52 for details.

Assessments
INITIAL EVALUATION DATE (WEEK 1):
MID-POINT EVALUATION DATE (WEEK 4):
SUMMARY EVALUATION DATE (WEEK 9):

FUNCTIONAL ASSESSMENT	COMPLETE (Yes/No)	DISCOMFORT (Yes/No)	NOTE DIFFICULTY
Overhead Squat			
Standing with Eyes Closed (two legs)			
Standing with Eyes Closed (one leg)			
Heel to Toe Walking			
Getting up from a Chair			

PHYSICAL FITNESS ASSESSMENT	GOAL	INITIAL	MID-POINT	SUMMARY
Chair Sit	1 Minute			
Push-up	20 Max			
Forward Plank	45 Secs			
Lateral Plank	45 Secs			
Six Minute Walk Test				
One Mile Walk Test				

Techniques

Reps: 10
Sets: 2
RPE: 5/10

Exercise	Page #	Equipment
Lifting Technique	66	weighted object
Rotating Technique	67	weighted object
Squatting Technique	68	chair

Posture Basics

Reps: 15
Sets: 1
RPE: 3/10

Exercise	Page #	Equipment
Hip Hinging	69	physio-ball
Spinal Whip	70	
Standing Tail Wag	71	
Thoracic Flex on Roller	72	foam roller or rolled towel
Shoulder Circles	73	foam roller or rolled towel

Self-Treatment and Massage

Reps: 15
Sets: 1
RPE: 2/10

Exercise	Page #	Equipment
Cranial Release	74	foam roller or rolled towel
Sacral Release	75	foam roller or rolled towel
Foam Roller Scissor Stretch	76	foam roller or rolled towel
MELT Ball Series	77	small ball

Mobility

Beginner Segment
Reps: 12
Sets: 1-2
RPE: 4/10

Exercise	Page #	Equipment
Ankle Pumps	87	rolled towel
Knee to Forehead	88	
Lateral Side Bend on Physio-ball	89	physio-ball, dowel or broom-stick
Physio-ball Roll	90	physio-ball
Draw the Sword/Return the Sword	91	physio-ball, weight (optional)

Intermediate Segment
Reps: 12
Sets: 1
RPE: 4/10

Exercise	Page #	Equipment
Hip Lifters	78	
Double Arm Stretch	79	two chairs or door frame
Wrist/Forearm Stretches	80	
Rotator Cuff Stretch	81	

Advanced Segment
Reps: 15
Sets: 2
RPE: 6/10

Exercise	Page #	Equipment
Double Arm Hug Rotation	82	chair
Alphabet Series (W's, Y's, T's)	83-85	chair
Ribcage Opener	86	foam roller or rolled towel

Balance

Beginner Segment
Reps/Seconds: 12
Sets: 1
RPE: 3/10

Exercise	Page #	Equipment
Assisted Rotational Chair Stretch	92	chair
Calf Raises	93	chair, foam roller or rolled towel
Heel to Toe Rocks	94	

Intermediate Segment
Reps/Seconds: 15
Sets: 2
RPE: 6/10

Exercise	Page #	Equipment
Heel to Toe Rocks	94	
Balancing on Half Roller	97	foam roller or rolled towel
Clock Series: Single Foot Touches (hold onto chair if needed)	96	chair (optional)

Advanced Segment
Reps: 12
Sets: 3
RPE: 7/10

Exercise	Page #	Equipment
Physio-ball Foot Lifts	95	physio-ball
Clock Series: Single Foot Touches	96	
Balancing on Half Roller	97	foam roller or rolled towel

Stability

Reps: 10
Sets: 2
RPE: 6/10

Exercise	Page #	Equipment
Kegel	98	physio-ball
All Fours Core Progression	99	
Chopping Movements	100	theraband, rolled towel
Lifting Movements	101	theraband, rolled towel
Single Reverse Kickback on Physio-ball	102	physio-ball

Strength

Beginner Segment
Reps: 12
Sets: 2
RPE: 6/10

Exercise	Page #	Equipment
Band Pulls	103	theraband, chair
Band Rows	104	theraband, chair
Front Pullbacks	105	theraband

Intermediate Segment
Reps: 10
Sets: 2-3
RPE: 7/10

Exercise	Page #	Equipment
Row with Tricep Extension	106	dumbbells
Band Presses with Two Arms	107	theraband, chair
Band Pulls with One Knee Up	108	theraband
Towel Pulls	109	chair, towel or blanket

Advanced Segment
Reps: 12
Sets: 3
RPE: 8/10

Exercise	Page #	Equipment
Row with Tricep Extension	106	dumbbells
Band Presses with Two Arms	107	theraband, chair
Band Pulls with One Knee Up	108	theraband
Band Rows	104	theraband, chair

Partner Workouts

Reps: 12
Sets: 1-2
RPE: 5/10

Exercise	Page #	Equipment
Chest Stretch Open Arms	110	chair
Shoulders/Torso Stretch	111	
Assisted Apley Stretch	112	
Double Hand Chest Press	113	
Single Hand Chest Press	114	
Weight Shifting	115	
Partner Stability Pushes	116	chair (optional)

Appendix

Your Healthy Brain Vision Statement

In the Healthy Brain Vision Statement, you'll write out goals and objectives as they relate to your patient's or loved one's mental and physical health.

For example, their doctor has told them that preventing falls, controlling high blood pressure, and engaging in regular mental activities will help in deterring mental and physical decline, and all of these are risk factors for dementia.

Break down these three factors into actionable steps that can be taken everyday. Here is an example: "On a daily basis I plan to practice balance exercises found in *Exercises for Brain Health,* keep my additive salt intake at a minimum, and journal my day-to-day activities."

Fill in your goals:
Mental Goals: _____

Physical Goals: _____

Fill in three objectives that you feel can be completed on a daily basis to help them achieve their goals above:

Mental Task: _____ (ex. write in journal)

Physical Task: _____ (ex. 15 minutes of exercise)

Social Task: _____ (ex. meet a new person)

Lifestyle Assessment

The questions below can be used by caregivers to help their patient or loved one in continuing to evaluate their goals and track their progress.

1. What are your main reasons for starting a fitness program (ex. weight loss, social, etc.)?

_____

_____

_____

_____

2. How would you describe your fitness condition in terms of your general health and fitness?

_____

_____

_____

_____

3. Have you ever done any structured exercise program? ☐ Yes ☐ No
If yes, please describe. (If no, please go to the next question)

_____

_____

_____

_____

How many times a week did you exercise? _____

How long did you continue the program?_____

Did you get the results you wanted? ☐ Yes ☐ No
If you did, why did you stop?

_____

_____

_____

_____

4. What activity do you enjoy doing the most?

_____

_____

_____

_____

5. What do you like doing the least?

_____

_____

_____

_____

6. What would you identify as the main barriers preventing you from exercising in the future?

☐ Procrastination ☐ Lack of motivation
☐ No time ☐ Lack of facilities
☐ Injury ☐ Lack of ability/fitness
☐ Financial cost ☐ Lack of relevant knowledge
☐ Family responsibilities ☐ Medical advice
☐ Intimidated

7. How many times per week are you willing to exercise?

_____

8. How long will you set aside each day? _____

9. How many units of alcohol do you drink in a typical week?
One unit of alcohol equals: ½ pint of standard beer/lager
                                 1 small glass of wine

10. Do you smoke? ☐ Yes ☐ No
How many do you smoke per day? _____
Do you want to stop smoking? ☐ Yes ☐ No

Goals
1. What health goals would you like to achieve in the next 3 months?

_____

_____

_____

2. What long-term health goals would you like to achieve over the next 12 months?

_____

_____

_____

_____

3. Name 3 things you will do in order to improve your health.

_____

_____

_____

_____

_____

_____

_____

_____

_____

_____

_____

_____

Testing Brain Function Under Stress

Throughout our daily activities our brain and body are placed under enormous amounts of stress. Each individual's body interprets stress in different ways. For example, running across the street may be considered extremely stressful for one person, while being asked to recall financial numbers at an important business meeting could be equally as stressful for another. So what's a fun, yet challenging, way to test our ability to function under cognitive stress?

The following can be an excellent tool for caregivers to measure regular cognitive health in patients or loved ones. Try creating your own version based upon the following guidelines:

1. Establish a quiet place where the patient can sit and relax for 5-10 minutes. Limit environmental stimuli including TV, reading excitable materials, phone calls, etc.

2. Take a baseline heart rate and blood pressure during this 10-minute quiet time.

3. Begin the exercise by counting back by 7's. For beginners (severe or diagnosed dementia), start at 100 and count backwards by 7 (100, 93, 86, etc.) For those with normal brain function, extend the test by beginning at 500 or 1000 and then count down.

4. Allow beginners a time frame of 3-5 minutes, and those with normal brain function as long as 10 minutes. This exercise seems simple but it may be stressful for those with advanced dementia or Alzheimer's.

5. Take heart rate and blood pressure every 2 minutes to measure stress response.

6. As the client or loved one becomes accustomed to the test, change it up with information that is important to daily function. For example, ask them to recite family members' phone numbers, addresses, grocery lists, banking/financial specifics, doctors' contact information, medicines, etc.

The point is to train the brain like a muscle: repetition, repetition, repetition! Enhance the efficiency of neural networks through repetitive actions.

Keeping the brain sharp with repetition of enjoyable activities is more important than any research that claims certain activities are better than others.

Examples of brain-building activities that they may enjoy include the following:
- Creating to-do lists
- Using calendars to make notes
- Watching enjoyable, stimulating TV shows or community events
- Setting a day to buy presents, gifts, or thoughtful items linked to dates on the calendar

Stress Survey

This Stress Survey can be helpful for caregivers in determining how dementia may be impacting the patient's stress levels. Help your patient or loved one fill out the following questions:

Section 1: Check off any of the following symptoms you have experienced in the past 30 days:
- ☐ Headaches/Migraines
- ☐ Digestive Trouble/Irregularity
- ☐ Irritability/Hormone Problems
- ☐ High Blood Pressure
- ☐ Sensitivity to Certain Foods
- ☐ Acid Reflux, Irritable Bowel Syndrome, Colitis, Hiatal Hernia, etc.
- ☐ Fatigue
- ☐ Nervousness
- ☐ Pain/Tension/Numbness
    - ☐ Neck
    - ☐ Legs
    - ☐ Shoulders
    - ☐ Arms
    - ☐ Low Back
    - ☐ Hands
- ☐ Sinus Problems/Allergies
- ☐ Weight Gain/Loss
- ☐ Arthritis
- ☐ Depression
- ☐ Insomnia/Sleep Problems
- ☐ Stress/Anxiety

Which of the above bothers you the most?

_____

How long have you been bothered by the condition?

_____

Describe how it feels or affects you when it is at its worst:

_____

_____

_____

Section 2: Does it cause you to be:
- [ ] Moody
- [ ] Irritable
- [ ] Sleepless
- [ ] Restricted from Daily Activities

Section 3: Does this affect your work through:
- [ ] Decision Making
- [ ] Poor Attitude
- [ ] Decreased Productivity
- [ ] Exhaustion
- [ ] Unable to work long hours

Section 4: Does this affect your personal life through:
- [ ] Losing patience with spouse or children
- [ ] Restricting ability to perform household duties
- [ ] Hindering ability to exercise or participate in sports
- [ ] Interfering with ability to participate/enjoy hobbies or other desired activities

Physical Activity Readiness Questionnaire

Help your patient or loved one fill out this questionnaire and present it to their primary care physician to assess their activity level and physical fitness before beginning an exercise program.

First Name _____ ☐ Male   ☐ Female

Last Name _____ Birth Date _____

Address _____ Height _____

City _____ State _____ Zip Code _____

Weight _____

Home Phone _____

Cell Phone _____

E-mail _____

1. ☐ Yes ☐ No Have you been inactive for the past 12 months?
2. ☐ Yes ☐ No Are you over age 65?
3. ☐ Yes ☐ No Has your doctor ever said you have a heart condition and recommended only medically supervised physical activity?
4. ☐ Yes ☐ No Do you have chest pains brought on by physical activity?
5. ☐ Yes ☐ No Have you ever experienced chest pains when not exercising?
6. ☐ Yes ☐ No Do you have high blood pressure?
7. ☐ Yes ☐ No Has a doctor ever recommended medication for your blood pressure or a heart condition?
8. ☐ Yes ☐ No Do you have elevated cholesterol levels?
9. ☐ Yes ☐ No Are you a Type II Diabetic?
10. ☐ Yes ☐ No Has your physician ever told you that you have a joint or bone problem that has been, or could be, made worse by exercise?
11. ☐ Yes ☐ No Do you feel dizzy/lose your balance/tend to lose consciousness?
12. ☐ Yes ☐ No Do you take prescribed drugs for health reasons?

List all drugs _____
_____
_____
_____

If you answered yes to one or more of the questions above, please answer the following questions:

13. ☐ Yes ☐ No Have you consulted your physician regarding increasing your physical activity and/or performing a fitness assessment?

14. ☐ Yes ☐ No If you answered no to question 8, will you contact your physician prior to increasing your physical activity and/or performing a fitness assessment?

Medical History: Please check all conditions that apply

☐ Heart Disease
☐ Stroke
☐ High Blood Pressure
☐ High Triglycerides
☐ Cancer
☐ Lung/Pulmonary Disease
☐ Kidney Disease
☐ Osteoporosis
☐ Ulcer
☐ Gastrointestinal Disease
☐ Depression
☐ Diabetes Mellitus (DM)
☐ Obesity
☐ Arthritis
☐ Rheumatoid arthritis
☐ Osteoarthritis
☐ Food Allergies
☐ Bulemia
☐ Anorexia
☐ Neuromuscular Disease
☐ Arteriosclerosis

☐ Psychological Problems
☐ Anemia
☐ Compulsive overeating disorder
☐ Low Back Pain
☐ Gallbladder Disease
☐ Diarrhea
☐ Pregnant/lactating or trying to conceive
☐ Currently being monitored or have been advised to be monitored by a physician
☐ Recommended high level care
☐ Special Diet
☐ Other medical condition (s) that may impact your fitness.
Explain _____
Any other medical problems:
_____
_____
_____
_____

Is there a family history of any of the following medical conditions?

☐ Heart problems   ☐ Diabetes
☐ Epilepsy   ☐ Early menopause
☐ Cancer   ☐ Other

If other, please explain:

_____

_____

_____

Have you had major surgery in the last 10 years?   ☐ Yes   ☐ No
If yes, please give details:

_____

Have you had minor surgery in the last 2 years?
If yes, please give details:

_____

_____

_____

Have you been diagnosed or treated by a physician or health professional for the following:

☐ Asthma   ☐ Heart Problems
☐ Epilepsy   ☐ Chest Pains
☐ High Blood Pressure   ☐ Other
☐ Diabetes   If other, please explain:

_____

_____

Do you ever experience the following symptoms?

☐ short of breath with very light exertion
☐ pain, pressure, heaviness or tightness in chest area
☐ regular unexplained pain in abdomen, shoulder, or arm
☐ severe dizzy spells or episodes of fainting
☐ regular lower leg pain during walking that is relieved by rest
☐ ever feel 'skips', palpitations or runs of fast beats in your chest

Do you have any of the following injuries?

☐ Knee/thigh injury   ☐ Shoulder injury   ☐ Nerve damage
☐ Back pain/injury   ☐ Head/Neck injury   ☐ Bone fracture
☐ Wrist/hand injury   ☐ Arm/Elbow injury
☐ Ankle/foot injury   ☐ Hip/pelvis injury

If you answered yes, please give details:

_____

_____

_____

Are these or any other injuries aggravated by exercise? ☐ Yes ☐ No
If yes, please give details:

_____

_____

_____

Are you presently receiving physical therapy? ☐ Yes ☐ No

Nutrition Tips and Recipes to Improve Brain Health

Recipes from *Navigating the Supermarket*, by William Smith and Christina Wellington, M.S.

Eating organically grown foods may help to improve health. Some research suggests that certain agricultural chemicals used in the conventional method of growing food may have the ability to cause genetic mutations that can lead to the development of cancer, as well as disrupt mitochondria function, which can inhibit the effectiveness of one's metabolism. Organic farms vary depending on their certification and practices, but most foster biological diversity and the health of the consumer, soil and environment. Instead of using harmful chemicals or bio-engineering, organic farms use natural methods, such as diversifying and rotating crops, and using natural fertilizer or cover crops to maximize soil fertility.

Organic foods are nutritionally superior to conventionally grown foods. This may sound like a bold statement, but the research proves it. Organic foods have been growing in popularity, not only in the United States, but worldwide. In 1998, a review of 34 studies comparing the nutritional content of organic versus non-organic food was published in *Alternative Therapies in Health and Medicine* (Volume 4, No. 1, pgs. 58-69). In this review, organic food was found to have "higher protein quality in all comparisons, higher levels of vitamin C in 58% of all studies, 5-20% higher mineral levels for all but two minerals." Organic foods also contain more flavonoids than conventionally grown foods, according to Danish research published in the August 2003 issue of the *Journal of Agricultural and Food Chemistry*.

When it comes to choosing between organic or conventionally grown foods, size doesn't matter. One study found that organically grown oranges contained up to 30% more vitamin C than those grown conventionally. The test group that ran this study expected that the conventionally grown oranges, which were twice as large, would have twice the vitamin C as the organic versions. However, the size ends up being much larger for the conventionally grown versions because, in conventional farming, nitrogen fertilizers are used. They cause an uptake of water, so this process dilutes the orange's flavor and nutritional value.

Eating organic may also help protect against inflammation, which for the average person, means a chance to age gracefully, a faster recover time for the athlete, as well as reduced risk for cancer, diabetes, and the prevention of other illnesses. Organic farming methods, which produce organic food, has also been seen as beneficial for aging gracefully by supplying the body with more antioxidants to fight against free radicals.

Recipes for a Healthy Brain

Baked Ziti

Ingredients:
2 cloves garlic
½ white or yellow onion, finely chopped
(cut down the center core, not horizontally)
½ lb. ground beef
1 (8oz.) jar tomato sauce
1 lb. whole-wheat Rigatoni
12 oz. low-fat Ricotta
Low-fat salsa

Directions:
Pre-heat oven to 375°.
Add garlic and onions to the pan and brown mixture on medium heat.
Brown ½ lb. ground beef in a separate pan, draining the fat juices.

Add ground beef to the garlic and onion mixture, and brown together.

Add tomato sauce to the beef, garlic, and onion mixture, then simmer on low heat for 10 minutes. Turn off heat and leave on oven surface.

Add1 lb. of Rigatoni to boiling water in a large pot and boil until tender.

Drain cooked Rigatoni and return to large pot, then add beef, garlic, and onion mixture to pot and mix gently.

Add low-fat Ricotta to beef and rigatoni mixture and mix thoroughly.

Move entire mixture into a casserole dish and spread evenly throughout the dish. Top with low-fat salsa.

Place casserole dish into pre-heated 375° oven for 25 minutes.

Turkey Pasta

Ingredients:
2 (8 oz.) turkey sausages
1 tsp. red pepper
7 leaves of kale, removed from stalk and chopped
½ onion
2 cloves garlic
1 lb. Penne pasta
1 (8 oz.) jar tomato sauce
Salt, to taste

Directions:
Sautee the turkey sausages, red pepper, and kale in olive oil over medium heat. Then add the onion and garlic. Simmer for 3 minutes.

Bring pasta to a boil, lightly salt to taste. Add tomato sauce to the first pan and stir on low heat. Pour the mixture over drained pasta.

Black Bean Stew with Turkey Sausage and Corn

This recipe requires a deep pan or a crockpot.

Ingredients:
½ clove garlic
½ onion (red or yellow)
1 tsp. red pepper (optional)
2 (8 oz.) turkey sausages, cut into slices
1 lb. corn
1 (28 oz.) can diced tomatoes
2 (8 oz.) cans black beans, undrained

Directions:
Simmer garlic and onion for 5 minutes. Add red pepper and turkey sausage, then simmer for 3 minutes. Add corn, diced tomatoes, and black beans, then simmer for 20 minutes on low heat.

Salmon Pasta

Ingredients:
½ onion
2 cloves garlic
1 (8 oz.) jar tomato sauce
1 lb. pink salmon
2 Tbsp. capers
4 Tbsp. black olives
1 lb. whole-wheat Fusilli

Directions:
Sautee onion and garlic, then add tomato sauce and cook for one minute on medium heat. Add salmon and cook for two minutes on medium heat. Add capers and black olives and simmer for 10 minutes.
Bring Fusilli to a boil, drain, and top with the prepared mixture.

Resources

Books

Genova, Lisa, *Still Alice.*

Mace, Nancy L., Peter V. Rabins, *The 36-hour Day: A Family Guide to Caring for People with Alzheimer Disease, Other Dementias, and Memory Loss in Later Life.*

Smith, William, Christina Wellington, *Navigating the Supermarket: A Nutritious Guide to Shopping Well.*

Websites

MedicineNet
www.medicinenet.com

WebMD
www.webmd.com

Organizations

Alzheimer's Association
www.alz.org

Alzheimer's Disease Education and Referral Center (ADEAR)
www.nia.nih.gov/Alzheimers

Centers for Disease Control and Prevention
www.cdc.gov

Eldercare Locator
www.eldercare.gov
800-677-1116 (toll-free)

National Institute of Aging
www.nia.nih.gov
800-222-2225 (toll-free)
800-222-4225 (TTY/toll-free)

National Institute of Neurological Disorders and Stroke
www.ninds.nih.gov

National Library of Medicine: Medline Plus
www.medlineplus.gov

NIH Senior Health
www.nihseniorhealth.gov

Parkinson's Alliance
www.parkinsonalliance.org

U.S. Department of Health and Human Services
www.hhs.gov

World Health Organization
www.who.int/en

Emergency Contact Information

Name _____ Relation _____

Address _____

City_____ State _____ Zip Code _____

Telephone: Home _____

                 Mobile _____

                 Work _____

Physician's Information

Name _____

Address _____

City _____ State _____ Zip Code _____

Telephone _____

31901047123130